Dedicated to my nephew

Ian Grzeskowiak

August 13, 1987 – February 19, 2007

Contents

Foreword by Dr. Rodney Ford

This book takes us on an improbable journey from catastrophic illness to gluten-free salvation. As Nadine states, "The truth is more frightening than any fiction." Hers is truly a frightening story about the terrible toll of undiagnosed gluten illness, especially in children. She has contemplated the horror of what would have happened to her had she not been diagnosed. Her frustrations, her compassion, and her future hopes can be felt on every page. Undoubtedly, you will also be left with a sense of frustration and bewilderment from Nadine's graphic descriptions of her decades of illness, her eventual diagnosis by a chance encounter, and her pathway to being fully healed. Perhaps the most distressing part of this book is to consider all of the still-suffering people who have yet to meet that someone who can understand and treat their illness. This is surely what has driven Nadine to tell her story.

I am a medical practitioner, with specialties in pediatrics, gastroenterology and allergy. I have spent my career looking after sick children, over which time I have discovered that the majority have become ill because of adverse reactions to what they are eating. Over thirty years ago, I began to investigate food allergies in children and witnessed that many children and their families got better when they quit gluten.

This observation spurred me on to research gluten-related illness, and I was a founder of the concept of "gluten syndrome," as well as one of the first to recognize that gluten was a neurotoxin. My medical practice, at the Children's Clinic and Allergy Centre, is in New Zealand. However, similar to many other countries, the possibility of celiac disease and gluten sensitivity causing chronic illness is seldom considered here. Globally, it seems that most medical practitioners remain uninformed about celiac disease and gluten-related disorders. This book will help remedy this deplorable state of affairs.

Nadine, a skilled emergency registered nurse, was forced on a long journey of self-discovery. For a long time, she was a lone voice. She was puzzled by the fact that in the 1950s, the condition "celiac disease" literally disappeared from the medical lexicon in the U.S., and that even in today's textbooks, celiac disease is considered a rare disease. She says that it seems as if celiac disease has been put in a time capsule which has yet to see the light of day.

Similar to Nadine, every day in my clinic I hear the frustrations of my patients, whose medical practitioners refuse to order the blood tests for celiac disease, and who ridicule the concept of gluten-related illnesses. This is despite rapidly accumulating scientific evidence documenting the huge disease burden caused by gluten consumption.

This is a family disease. We are predisposed to gluten harm through our genes. As Dr. Judith Stern once said, "Genetics loads the gun but the environment pulls the trigger." This exemplifies the complex relationship between human disease and the environment. Thankfully, a genetic test is available so that we can come to grips with our likelihood of gluten illness. But family members are frequently in denial about the possibility of gluten causing them harm. The idea that a food we crave could be making us ill is a truth that is hard to swallow. But gluten does cause multiple organ disease, especially in the gut, in the skin, and in the nervous system. Research now indicates that our nerves and brains are the main targets of this gluten harm.

Like Nadine, I too have been witness to the extreme reluctance of medical practitioners to recognize that foods can cause illness. But it turns out that just about any food can cause allergic/intolerance reactions. At least a quarter of the population has some sort of food reaction, and gluten has now been recognized as the number-one harmful food. However, the prevalence of gluten-related illness has yet to be properly documented. Nadine takes us through the historical details of these diseases, and their emergence over the past decade in the U.S. She explains that gluten cannot be properly digested by the human gastrointestinal tract, that it causes inflammation in our intestines, that it can trigger many autoimmune diseases, and that it causes an amazingly wide range of illnesses that are usually attributed to other conditions.

Most gastroenterologists view celiac disease as a condition limited to the mucosa. And most dermatologists view dermatitis herpetiformis as a condition limited to the skin. This could not be further away from the truth. When you read this book, you will be astonished by the far-ranging symptoms of gluten diseases. Hence, Nadine's impassioned plea for anybody with any chronic ailment to be tested for celiac disease, and to consider the possibility of gluten intolerance. As Nadine says, dermatitis herpetiformis is merely an expression of what is happening deep down your body. So, if you have a chronic rash, then you also have damage in other organs as well. Likewise, if you have inflammation in your gut, then you will also have inflammation elsewhere. Consequently, everyone needs testing.

But there is a conundrum. Although everybody should be tested for celiac disease, the standard available tests are not very accurate. The celiac tests (most commonly the IgA tissue transglutaminase antibody, or tTG-IgA) will not accurately pick up early celiac disease, and gives no clues that could lead to a diagnosis of gluten intolerance. Additionally, most people suffering from gluten harm will have a normal endoscopy result, a test that is the current mainstay of gastroenterological investigations of gut damage from gluten.

So diagnosis is difficult! It turns out that the only surefire way to work out if gluten is harming you is to adopt a gluten-free lifestyle for at least a year and watch for any benefits. When I say "gluten-free," I would be more accurate to tell you to go "gluten-zero." This is because even tiny amounts of gluten can continue to trigger inflammation. You will not heal if residual gluten remains in your diet.

Already, a third of the North American population has chosen to adopt a gluten-free lifestyle, and this is testament to how commonly gluten harm is being experienced. But it is likely that the grain manufacturers will not be sympathetic to this gluten-zero movement. It is likely that medical practitioners will be reluctant to accept the concept of widespread gluten harm. It is likely that the pharmaceutical industry will continue to urge doctors to prescribe drugs to treat symptoms that simply stem from adverse gluten reactions. It is likely that celiac researchers will want to develop vaccines and drugs to combat gluten harm. And it is likely that doctors like me, and nurses like Nadine, will continue to be ostracized by our colleagues for pointing out the common symptoms caused by gluten.

However, we have hope. We have seen countless gluten sufferers who have followed our path: from gluten victim to gluten-free advocate. As more and more people like us understand the terrible toll of disease caused by eating gluten, a whole new way of eating will be adopted. The first step of going gluten free is just the beginning. Nadine urges us to tell others about our own experiences, and to vote with our gluten-free dollars.

Dr. Rodney Ford, MD, MBBS, FRACP

www.drrodneyford.com

Author of *The Gluten Syndrome: Is Wheat Causing You Harm?*
(www.glutensyndrome.com),
Gluten Brains: the brain-grain connection
(www.glutenbrains.com), and
Gluten Related Disorder: Sick? Tired? Grumpy?
(www.glutenrelateddisorder.com)

Acknowledgements

After going through the entire process of writing a book, I have complete and total respect for anyone who has ever written a book, ever. It takes a fair amount of tenacity and fortitude to get to the finished product: an actual book. I would like to thank everyone, everywhere who has contributed to this book in whatever capacity. I have a core group of people around me who are incredibly loving, supportive, and encouraging, and these are the people I am very grateful for in my life. I would also like to congratulate the people who have recognized they have the power to choose what they consume and to change the world by making educated decisions, thinking critically, recognizing a sick person, and acting appropriately.

Dough Nation

Nothing to Do with What You're Eating

I stepped out of the shower one day in October 2006, looked in the mirror, and gave myself six months to live. I was forty years old and I prayed it wouldn't take me six months to die. I felt like a ninety-plus-year-old woman, and I now have complete and total empathy for people who are just done living. I even smelled like a dying person.

I tried to explain my situation to one of my oldest friends from high school, Alison. I told her I smelled like I was rotting from the inside out. She looked disgusted and then said, "If I ever smell like that, will you tell me? Promise?"

My hair was falling out. My eyes were bugging out of my head. I looked like Marty Feldman. Not good. I had canker sores in my mouth, which my mother always told us was caused by using swear words. My arms and legs were numb, especially the fourth and fifth digits on both my hands and my feet. My doctors had suggested the numbness was due to the fact I was a knitter, and I reminded them that I didn't knit with my feet. I had intermittent chest pain and premature ventricular contractions, which was disconcerting for a forty-year-old woman who also happened to be a certified emergency nurse specializing in trauma and critical care. I had fluid in my lungs most of the time. At any given time during the day, I looked like I was between three and nine months pregnant. Thank God for stretchy pants and scrubs.

All my muscles and joints hurt. I weighed forty pounds more than I do now. I had 4+ pitting edema, which I lovingly referred to as my "Eastern European Potato-Picking Legs" My ninety-two-year-old grandmother had them too, so I just figured I had inherited that particular trait. Plus, I tried to rationalize that I worked twelve-hour shifts on a concrete floor, so why wouldn't my ankles be retaining fluid like water balloons? But, I noted, many of the other nurses' ankles weren't edematous at the end of their twelve-hour shifts. Also, my lymph nodes were swollen in my chest and in my left armpit. At one point, I thought I had a cyst, or an ingrown hair or something in my left armpit and tried to drain it myself. Not a good idea, and I would not recommend you try that at home, because if it is a swollen lymph node, they tend to bleed. A lot.

As if that wasn't enough, I also had this hellacious rash. I always, and I do mean always, had eczema. As a redhead, I was told I should just to expect to have sensitive skin. For many years, I was considered a hippie because I didn't shave my armpits or my legs, because it would cause my skin to break out and be "sensitive." This was misdiagnosed as many different things. I saw so many dermatologists over the years, and was prescribed tubes and tubes of prescription steroid creams and lotions and special soaps. None of them helped. Most of my relatives also had this rash, so we all thought it was another one of those familial traits that we all just "had." My grandmother related stories of putting Preparation H on her hands to relieve the itching (since it contains hydrocortisone cream). For years and years, my hands were red, swollen, cracked, bleeding, and itchy, and I frequently had teeny, tiny blisters between my fingers just underneath the skin. It was embarrassing. The only thing that relieved the pain and itching was running my hands under super-HOT tap water for as long as I could stand it. The dermatologists all agreed that was not helpful, but I did it anyway. During one of the flare-ups, one of the older nurses I was working with at the time suggested I had scabies. It wasn't scabies, but I lost a night of sleep until I could confirm it the next day.

That rash on my hands frequently got worse when I was at work, so I thought I was allergic to latex gloves. I only bought cotton underwear and bras. I wore cotton gloves to bed. My skin itched. When I was younger, I thought I was allergic to metals because my ear lobes would get crusty and ooze when I wore earrings, so I stopped wearing earrings. Under my bra, and on my scalp and legs I would get transient, intermittent patches of painfully itchy skin, sometimes with a rash and sometimes not. One day, the rash disappeared from my hands and started exploding on other areas of my body. A linear rash on the inside of my left thigh, behind my knees and my elbows, on my right anterior lower leg, on the top of my foot, and all over my torso, plus two special patches at the top of my butt cheeks. I lovingly referred to this particularly irritating, painful and intensely itchy patch as my "ass rash." My eyelids, lips and face would get dry, scaly, wrinkly, and itchy, along with painful monthly breakouts of acne that seemed rather deep and cystic. My skin was not my friend.

As I was deciding whether to call to get admitted to hospice or just keep working (I would have just kept working—I'm Polish), I realized it would be bad if I died for my daughter, Hannah, who was ten years old at the time. So I tried to self-diagnose. I read every dermatology book ever written. I researched my symptoms. I figured someone had to know what was wrong with me. But despite having what I as a nurse considered REAL symptoms, it had been suggested by some of the doctors that I was "faking" things. To be sure, on paper I looked great. I was chronically mildly anemic, which had also been suggested by many doctors was because I have red hair, which is not based in any science. My thyroid tests were all negative. Based on my lab work alone, I did "look great," but clinically, my body was a mess. They referred me to psychologists and psychiatrists. They prescribed me medications—a grocery bag full by the time I was done. None of those prescription medications made me better, and I am pretty sure most of them made me worse.

In my quest to have an official diagnosis and find out what was killing me, I made appointments with doctors who were outside of my work venue. I considered this to be against my "religion" and not the optimal way to spend my time when I wasn't working. As children, we were raised to *not* go to the doctor unless we were dying or at least bleeding profusely. As a medically minded person, I would ask the different doctors I would see very pointed questions. I wanted to be a "good" patient and be involved in my health care. I would ask things like, "Hey, do you think I might have AIDS or hepatitis? I am at risk for those working in the emergency department (ED). Do you think I might have a brain tumor? I've lost my senses of taste and smell." When I lost those senses, I figured I just might as well be dead. Those doctors would reassure me that I didn't have those things, and most never even bothered to offer to test me for anything. They would just offer to write me more prescriptions for the symptoms, or as we like to call them in the emergency department, party favors.

I also seemed quite susceptible to sinus infections, even as a child, but much more so as an adult. My nose would run. I would sneeze, a lot. There were always several boxes of tissues in my house, the car and little packages for travel or hankies. My sinuses got to be such an issue that I would go to sleep with tissues tucked under my nose or stuffed up into my nasal cavities. During the night, the constant nasal congestion or sinusitis seemed to clear somewhat, but each morning I would feel as if I were experiencing an avalanche inside my head, and then I would start sneezing uncontrollably. I referred to this phenomenon as my sneeze alarm. Once it started, I was never able to go back to sleep. I saw allergists and ear, nose and throat doctors. I had skin tests that showed I was allergic to dust and dust mites. WHAT? That did not seem to make much sense to me. Thank goodness I drew the line and didn't buy all of those mattress and pillow covers and cases. What I remember is becoming an Afrin junkie, and using and abusing nasal spray morning and night. I would blow and blow my nose but nothing significant ever really came out. That was frustrating. I could feel all of this congestion and drainage, but moving it out was not happening. I became convinced I had either a truffle or a troll that lived in my right maxillary sinus. It hurt, and nothing would make it better or go away. I bought more and more over-the-counter sinus medications, herbal tinctures, sprays, and treatments, all to no avail.

I was seeing an ENT doctor at this time who suggested nasal surgery that would involve placing balloons in my sinus drainage holes, blowing up the balloons in an effort to create bigger holes (in my head!) so that the sinuses would drain. The doctor said he had small balloons and large balloons, but had never used the large balloons. I requested that he use the large balloons. A cut-to-the-chase solution, or so I thought.

But the reality was that I did not have a drainage issue. I had an inflammation issue. Even the biggest holes in my head would not have solved or resolved my sinus issues. I had to learn the hard way that gluten and dairy were causing the inflammation in my sinuses and in my respiratory system. No gluten and no dairy, including butter and ghee, no inflammation. Simple. But I had to find that out myself. Otherwise my only options were more steroids or another surgery, as I had been told by a different ENT doc.

Seriously, I would use the Neti pot and the salt water would never go through! There was no flushing occurring. My sinuses were so swollen and inflamed that I could barely breathe at times. The two events that frightened me occurred in the shower. I was taking a shower to inhale the steam in an effort to clear my sinuses. What happened on these two occasions was that the inflammation had become so bad, I could not swallow! I could not swallow at all. Apparently, one needs sinuses to be semi-operational for the pressure changes that allow for the physical act of swallowing. Torture. I had to emergently call the ENT doctor to meet me at his office so he could spray something up my nose to alleviate the swelling so I could swallow! I asked him if this could be caused by something I was eating.

His unequivocal answer: "No, It has nothing to do with what you are eating."

I would soon come to know just how wrong he was.

Suffering in the Bowels of History

There is a kind of chronic indigestion which is met with in persons of all ages, yet is especially apt to affect children between one and five years old. Signs of the disease are yielded by the fœces; being loose, not formed, but not watery; more bulky than the food taken would seem to account for; pale in colour, as if devoid of bile; yeasty, frothy, an appearance due to fermentation; stinking, stench often very great, the food having undergone putrefaction rather than concoction.

{....}

The causes of the disease are obscure. Children who suffer from it are not all weak in constitution. Errors in diet may perhaps be a cause, but what error? Why, out of a family of children all brought up in much the same way, should one alone suffer? This often happens.

{....}

Naked-eye examination of dead bodies throws no light upon the nature of the coeliac affection: nothing unnatural can be seen in the stomach, intestines or other digestive organs.

{....}

The onset is usually gradual, so that its time is hard to fix: sometimes the complaint sets in suddenly, like an accidental diarrhœa; but even when this is so, the nature of the disease soon shows itself.

—from Samuel Gee's "On the Cœliac Affection" (1888)

Wheat is ubiquitous in our culture. It is in our national song of pride, our amber waves of grain. It is well represented in the Bible as both wheat and bread, and is used in religious ceremonies to represent the body of Christ. Wheat is embossed in the carpet and prominently displayed in the artwork of the Oregon State capitol building. It is in our food, makeup, lotions, Play-Doh, glue in envelopes and stamps, in our compostable eating utensils, plates, and cups, our artwork, holiday wreaths, and business logos, and even our toilet paper (eeek!).

Celiac disease, meanwhile, has been in the medical history books forever. It was first named *koiliakos,* meaning "suffering in the bowels," by the Aretaeus of Cappadocia, who lived in ancient Greece in the second century A.D. In 1888, Dr. Samuel Gee, a British pediatrician, referred to it as "The Coeliac Affection" in his study of the condition, which he also recognized in adults. Dr. Gee put affected children on special diets, but because he was unsure of what caused the condition in the first place, the diets unfortunately included lightly toasted bread and those children died.

From 1908 to 1924, an American pediatrician, Dr. Sidney V. Haas, and his son, Dr. Merrill P. Haas, developed the specific carbohydrate diet or SCD in an effort to heal these children. Together they also wrote the book *Management of Celiac Disease,* published in 1951. Bananas were the primary source of carbohydrates on the Haas diet, and so these children became known as the "banana children." An article in the *New York Times* dated October 4, 1942, reported a banana shortage and documented how the doctors were treating the "children with celiac with injections of large doses of crude liver extract and vitamin B complex given on alternate days. The article went on to note that "[c]onsiderable improvement took place within three to six weeks, instead of an average of two years by the older treatment."

Management of Celiac Disease is a fascinating source book for anyone who is interested in the history of celiac disease. The pediatricians that were investigating celiac disease in the early 20th century, from roughly 1890 through to 1952, dabbled in various theories and trafficked in numerous treatments for the condition. The focus of these doctors' research and the nature of their approach to treatment was at times eerily on target and at other times wholeheartedly missed the target, in hindsight. But celiac disease was very much on their radar.

It was not until shortly after the end of World War II that Dr. Willem Dicke, a Dutch pediatrician, was credited with determining "gluten" as the component in grains that was making children sick and die. Before the war, when grains were readily available and people ate lots of bread, the children were sick and no one could figure out why. During the war, though, with cereal grains unavailable, and starvation a very real issue, the resourceful Dutch turned to tulip bulbs to make flour and bread. During those lean years, the sick children stopped dying, and in fact regained their health.

Soon after the war ended, grains were back on Dutch tables, and those same children became sick again. Their mothers went to Dr. Dicke and reported that the children had gotten healthy, even during a period of starvation, but now that the grains were back in their diets, those children were getting sick again and appeared to be starving.

One of my favorite Internet finds is an article in the *New York Times* dated May 21, 1950, entitled "'Celiac Disease': Most Children Are Now Cured But Cause Is Still Unknown." The article recounts a meeting of specialists in children's diseases of the New York University–Bellevue Medical Center in conjunction with the Society for Pediatric Research and the American Pediatric Society. The article discusses how Dr. Haas gave his children what his colleagues in pediatrics regarded as dangerous amounts of fats, and the children throve on it. Said the article, "Sixty years ago celiac disease was incurable and often even fatal. Today cures are certain in over 90 percent of the cases, and deaths are rare." This was in 1950.

But as the decade progressed, Europe and the United States began to take divergent paths with celiac disease. Shortly after the *New York Times'* coverage of the disease in 1950 and the publication of *Management of Celiac Disease* the following year, celiac disease remarkably disappeared from the medical literature in the U.S., and little or no research was done after 1952. The same paragraphs from medical textbooks in the 1950s can be found virtually verbatim in American medical textbooks as late as 2008, usually stating that celiac disease in the United States is incredibly rare, at a rate of 1 in 5,000 or even 10,000.

So what happened that celiac disease literally "disappeared" in this country for well over sixty years? The government was concerned about starvation. World War II had just ended and there was a population explosion—the baby boom. Our government was concerned about how all of these people were going to get fed. So it was decided—in my mind in a smoky back room somewhere—that the United States was going to start growing wheat, corn, soy, peanuts, potatoes, rice, and a few other primary protein sources, and they were going to grow a lot of them.

I would like to think someone, maybe a farmer, in one of these meetings might have said something like, "Hey what about all of the people who can't eat wheat because of celiac disease and gluten intolerance?" And what I am fairly certain occurred was the following response: "We know some people are going to get sick, and some people are going to die. But for the greater good, this is our plan and we are going ahead with it."

Because that's what they did. And it's how the United States still practices agriculture today.

Running Out of Gas

My plummet into multi-system organ failure started in January 2003. I was driving to Newport (Oregon) Hospital to work a thirty-six-hour weekend in the emergency department. The drive takes an hour from door to door, and I was making good time. My car heater was on but not on high, and I was dressed normally. But as I was flipping through the radio stations, I realized I was feeling warm. This was odd in itself, because I rarely felt warm. Even in the summer, I would wear turtlenecks and thick wool socks because I was always cold. Of course, I knew I had Raynaud's syndrome-slash-disease-slash-phenomenon, and my hands were for the most part purple, with a capillary refill time of more than twenty seconds. When I was younger and not a nurse, I had thought my hands were purple because I grew up in Buffalo, where it is always bone-chillingly cold, except when it was hot and muggy. My friends in the ED had been instructed NOT to use my capillary refill as an indicator that I needed to be intubated.

When I arrived for my shift in the ED, I stuck in the ear thermometer and pressed the button, and the machine arrived at a temperature of 102.4 degrees Fahrenheit. Surely the thermometer was broken. I tested it again with a different one. Nope, still 102.4. The other nurses and I laughed. I felt fine, not sick in the least. As a matter of fact, I had never missed a day of work due to illness. I always showed up and worked. I rarely took a day off except for vacations, and I never went home early from a shift due to illness. I thought I had a super immune system because of all of the interesting "stuff" I had been exposed to working in emergency departments over all those years. And because I felt fine and we could not find a source of the fever, I stayed and worked. We dipped my urine, which was negative for infection, and my nurse friends and the docs listened to or auscultated my lungs, but they couldn't hear anything odd. Strange.

By the middle of my third twelve-hour shift, I started to feel just a wee bit funky. I signed myself out and drove home to Corvallis. I took two Tylenol and went to bed, because that is what nurses do.

In the morning, when I woke up, I felt the worst I have ever felt in my life. Bad. Horrible. I felt so bad I was crying, which I don't make a habit of doing, even in the worst of circumstances. My whole body was racked by pain and I was shaking uncontrollably. My kids, Rory and Hannah, were in school and my then-husband, Brad, was working a twenty-four-hour shift at the fire station, so I drove the very short distance to immediate care, where I had worked as a medical assistant while I was still in school earning my RN. I was sobbing in the waiting room, and not in a quiet way. The sound and sight of me seemed to be frightening the other patients, because they all gave me a wide berth. I was scaring *myself,* for Pete's sake. I was escorted back to an exam room, where my vitals were taken and I was advised to put on a gown.

Thankfully, my friend Dr. Takush was on duty that day. He looked concerned when he walked in and saw me sobbing like a mad woman. He ordered a chest x-ray and had some blood drawn. I waited and sobbed some more, by myself. Dr. Takush opened the door, brought me out to the viewing box, and clipped in my x-ray. The reason we couldn't hear my pneumonia was because it was an atypical perihilar pneumonia that sat in my mid-right chest. Levaquin, a very potent fluoroquinolone antibiotic was prescribed, as it was the standard of care for hospital-acquired pneumonia (HAP) and community-acquired pneumonia (CAP). For many, many reasons, I no longer recommend people take any potent fluoroquinolone antibiotics unless they absolutely have to. This particular class of antibiotic is considered "broad spectrum," and it acts like a carpet bomb, taking out all of your good bacteria along with the bad.

My pneumonia seemed to get better, but I quickly developed a systemic yeast infection, which most unpleasantly caused me to develop vaginal and rectal fissures. Ouch. From that point on, my health began to plummet out of control. The next almost four years were spent seeing doctors outside of work. I would see internal medicine or family practice doctors and ask all sorts of questions about my symptoms and possible diseases. The standard answer seemed to be, "Gee, I don't know what's wrong with you, but here's a prescription for antibiotics." Or for prednisone. Or nasal sprays. Or Atarax. Or Ativan. Or lotions. Or for more and more antibiotics.

The list goes on and on. Some of the medications seemed to help for a day or two, but never longer. And the rebounds were getting to be noticeably worse each time.

The lymph node in my left armpit also became more swollen and tender. This seemed to coincide with a large mass in my left breast between two and three o'clock. I also had a large, deep, very painful rash right in that same area. My breasts had always been described as fibrous or lumpy, but this was clearly different. So I made an appointment with the best boob doctor in the area, one my nurse friends had also seen and deemed worthy. I went in, and he examined my breasts and said he didn't think it was breast cancer. Great. But if it turned out to be breast cancer, I had decided to go ahead and have a double mastectomy. My motto has always been to cut to the chase. If one of my breasts had to go, take both of them at the same time. He walked out of the room and didn't come back. I eventually got dressed and walked out. Okay, then.

It was also during this period of time that I realized my soul was disappearing. I have mentioned this phenomenon to a few other people who were really sick before they were diagnosed celiac or simply went gluten free, and they understand what I am talking about. I would drive around town and contemplate where my personality, my humor, and my very being were disappearing to. I had lost the very essence of my being, and this was very disconcerting to me. My mental picture of myself was like a Picasso painting where all of the facial and body parts are misshapen and distorted. Was I going mad? Is this what that feels like? I literally felt as if I had lost my mind and my soul. And if my soul was dying, was this a foreshadowing of my physical body dying?

So instead of hospice, in a last-ditch effort, I called one of the only dermatologists I hadn't seen, Dr. Abigail Haberman, making yet another appointment with a doctor outside of work, which was still against my religion, but had become somewhat of a bad habit in my quest to find what was killing me.

So I found myself in another doctor's office, in nothing but a threadbare gown, sitting on another exam table. In addition to the symptoms above, I explained to Nurse Helen that I also had profuse night sweats, my muscles and joints hurt, my hair was falling out, my eyes were horribly dry, and I was forty pounds overweight with what I called "crap fat" that wouldn't go away no matter what I did—along with my very attractive 4+ pitting edema. I had what felt like a brick in my belly even though I only ate small portions. I had just had sinus surgery that month that did not relieve any of my chronic, unrelenting, almost complete sinus congestion. After telling Nurse Helen all of the symptoms I could remember, she left the room and Dr. Haberman came in.

"I know what you have," Dr. Haberman said to me. "You have celiac disease and dermatitis herpetiformis. It's really rare and I have never diagnosed it before, but that's what you have."

To which I responded, "I have been a nurse for 14 years and I have no idea what you just said. I have what?"

She responded, "It means you can't eat gluten."

"Okay. What's gluten?" I asked.

"Gluten is wheat, barley, rye, and oats. You can't eat gluten anymore."

I was both excited and petrified at the same time. I said, "Okay, but I eat wheat, barley, rye, and oats for breakfast, lunch, and dinner. Plus, depending on how my shift goes in the emergency department, I might have a beer or two..."

"You can't do that anymore," she responded. "We are going to do a blood test and a skin biopsy today to confirm the diagnosis. After the blood is drawn, go immediately on a gluten-free diet."

Dr. Haberman is very efficient. She drew my blood and did two punch biopsies from the top of my right butt cheek, near my ass rash.

I went home, still excited and still petrified. I told my family I have a really rare disease and I can't eat anymore. I just can't, because I have this really rare disease and this is why I have the rash and all of the other symptoms, and if I go on this very specific diet, I will get better. They looked at me like I was completely crazy.

I went to the computer and punched in celiac disease and gluten. I was shocked that there was actually information on my really rare disease, and other people had it too! That was a relief right there. I printed off some information and started eating what I thought was gluten free, based on my limited knowledge and what the Internet told me. We cleaned out the cupboards. We vacuumed them, scrubbed, vacuumed again, and scrubbed again. Brad and I went shopping. We found a few shelves at Fred Meyer that had gluten-free products to replace the gluten-containing ones, things like pasta, crackers, bread, and all of those other foods I had eaten my whole entire life without, I thought, any problem before now.

I refer to this period of time as my "deer in the headlights" period, during which I was still, as I like to say, gluten addle-brained. It's not a surprise that I was gluten addle-brained for a while after quitting gluten cold turkey, because I was a gluten junkie. No kidding, and I am completely serious. I had a loaf of artisanal bread, instead of the proverbial monkey, on my back all the time. It was riding around with me every day and I had no idea.

I was a *functional* gluten junkie, mind you, but there were lots of signs I had a problem. I was committed to breads and pastries and anything made with grains. The number one thing I would seek out as I traveled was always the BEST bakery. Admittedly, I was never a big pie or cake eater; I certainly would eat them if they were readily available or in celebration of someone's birthday or wedding. But there were probably not many days in my whole life when I did not inoculate myself with wheat or grains in some form, usually starting off in the morning with toast, oatmeal, a bagel or two, or wheat germ added to my smoothie, because it was super good for me and my health and I was of course interested in my health and being healthy.

Plus, I suffered from constipation. I was frequently FOS or full of shit, literally and figuratively. I would eat oatmeal, bran muffins, cream of wheat, wheat germ, and anything that was suggested to be high in fiber. I was told my constipation would be better if I just ate MORE fiber. Constipation is not a lack-of-fiber issue; it is a neurological issue. The vagus nerve runs from your brain to your intestines. If your intestines are damaged, so are your intestinal nerves, and your intestines cannot perform the task referred to as peristalsis, which is the smooth muscle movement that pushes fecal material through your intestines on its way to the toilet. I was constipated due to neurological damage.

I also remember, as I am certain my friends and family members do, times when I would go into the bathroom and stay there for a good long while. This even happened on an airplane once. High altitudes were not my friend. My guts would blow up like a potato chip bag and I would either feel like I had to pass a watermelon, or that I would just succumb to the pressure and explode. Hanging out in your bathroom at home with magazines and music and potpourri is one thing, but trying to pass gas, a turd, or anything at 30,000 feet in the one toilet available in coach will piss off most if not all of the other waiting passengers. Try to imagine walking out of the cubicle toilet into that narrow aisle and excusing yourself and your bloated potato-chip-bag belly to a line of pissed-off people thirteen deep. Especially after you haven't passed anything but twenty minutes of time on your flight to Chicago. I was pissed too.

Every year for almost twenty years now, a group of emergency department friends, paramedics, and assorted others would gather for three days and two nights at Silcox Hut on Mount Hood. Silcox Hut is a ski lodge that sits a mile above Timberline Lodge on Mount Hood and is exquisite in its location, timber-hewn architecture, and unpretentious, exclusive coziness. There were only a few years I was unable to attend this yearly event, and I believe those years I missed will be what I regret on my deathbed. I could write a whole other book about the shenanigans and escapades that occurred there and the riotous times we experienced.

Prior to my diagnosis of celiac disease by accident, I still drank beer and ate gluten at this yearly event. As a matter of fact, I drank a fair amount of beer, as we all did, whilst playing poker or cribbage. One of my dear (asshole) friends (Hi, Joe!) and I would joyously engage in burping and farting contests, and some years it was super hard to tell who actually won, we were both that good at producing gas. We were both very talented and gifted in eructing/belching. One year, I was bunking with a critical care nurse, Kelly, at 14,000 feet, and apparently during the night, I passed a fair amount of aforementioned gas, unbeknownst to me. Kelly loudly exclaimed to my fellow emergency comrades the next morning that there was something seriously wrong with me. If she had to bunk with me, in the future, she was bringing a gas mask. She never came to another Silcox Hut event after that, at least not that I saw.

It is at this time that I would like to take a moment and apologize to Kelly. I wasn't being trying to be malicious or taint all of the useable oxygen in the lodge. And it is cold outside, sometimes there's a snowstorm, and it's dark. Running for your life and/or oxygen in the middle of the bona fide mountain is generally discouraged. If an emergency, trauma, or critical care nurse or doctor thinks there may be something wrong with you, someone should plan to stage an intervention and try to FIND OUT WHY THAT PERSON, A FRIEND AND COLLEAGUE, IS PASSING ENOUGH GAS OUT THEIR ASS TO CLEAR A HIGH-ALTITUDE SKI LODGE (unbeknownst to said person). Generally speaking, not intervening is unacceptable.

Initially, during my deer-in-the-headlights period when I was still gluten addle-brained and beginning to detox from forty years of being poisoned by my food, I did the basics. I went on a kick-starter elimination diet that ended up with me eating lots of cruciferous vegetables such as broccoli, kale, cabbage, cauliflower, and Brussels sprouts, raw green leafies like spinach, and fresh apples and pears. I did this for ten-day stretches at least twice. I used detox products and drank lots of water. We cleaned out our kitchen and restocked it with gluten-free flours and whole grain teff and quinoa. We all cooked and baked gluten-free muffins. Brad, always a pie master, perfected his gluten-free piecrust so that people preferred his gluten-free pies to the ones made with wheat flour. The crusts were amazingly light and flaky. He even taught several gluten-free pie baking classes in our home. We were getting good at eating gluten free as a family, at least at home.

During this time, I ate an enormous amount of food, and I still lost thirty-five pounds without even trying. All of the edema, bloating, and "crap fat" just seemed to disappear. I ate and ate and ate all of the gluten-free food I could get my hands on. It was at this point my family declared they probably couldn't keep me much longer because I was eating too much food. The fact was, my body had been starving of nutrients for a very long time, despite eating what I thought was very good, nutritious food, based on what I had been taught. We didn't eat fast food. We didn't have too many sugary snacks or frozen, prepared foods in our house. But because of the damage to my intestines, even if I had been eating nutritious foods, as long as I was still poisoning my body with wheat and other grains, my body would not be able to absorb any of those nutrients.

What I now know is that I was duped into thinking the food we were eating was the best food possible for me and my family. I had no idea that the bread, pasta, wheat flour, and oats that we were consuming at every meal were the cause of my lifelong symptoms and my plummet into multi-system organ failure.

Chronic stomach issues, pain. Constipation for as long as I remember.

Back on Tract

Your digestive system starts in your mouth and ends at your anus. This tube is about twenty-five to thirty feet long and is initially like a steep water slide that empties into a pool of stomach acid. In your mouth, your food gets chewed up and mixed with enzymes that begin the process of breaking down the food into smaller components so the nutrients can be absorbed and eventually utilized by the cells of the body. The food hits your stomach acid, also known as hydrochloric acid, which should be a pH of between 1 and 2—very acidic. The acid liquefies the food you just ate, and ideally kills any bacteria, viruses, or parasites in it. The food then gets squirted out through the pylorus into the duodenal bulb, then into the duodenum, jejunum, ileum, and colon, and the waste products finally get excreted through the rectum. Throughout the entire GI tract, vitamins, minerals, proteins, and all of the good nutrition is allowed into the blood system via what acts—in a healthy gut—like a lock-and-key system.

This is the abridged version of eating/digestion/pooping. This whole process that our body completes every time we eat is remarkably complex yet very efficient in a healthy person. We eat food, the food gets digested, our body takes the nutrients it needs to keep healthy and working, and we poop/excrete out the waste that is not helpful and possibly harmful to our body. It is a task that almost every human being who has ever lived is very good at performing.

That said, it is also a process that is susceptible to breaking down or malfunctioning based on our genetics, the foods we eat, and other environmental factors. Our bodies are remarkable at compensating for errors in judgment regarding food choices, but typically only for so long. At some point, most of us reach a tipping point into unwellness. We may gently slide into that unwellness with many small indicators that we are headed on the wrong path, but often we ignore these signs, take over-the-counter medications, or—if the symptoms become bad enough—we seek out a medical practitioner to prescribe medications to "fix" what ails us or at least quell those annoying symptoms that are interfering with our activities of daily life. Or for some of us, our bodies compensate for a very long time until there is a trigger event into the plummet stage of profound ill health or even straight to death.

As human beings, we do not have the enzymes to break down the proteins in wheat, barley, rye, and oats. When we eat the gluten protein, in any form, it either passes through our digestive tract and doesn't cause any damage, or it acts as a trigger for either inflammation (in the case of gluten intolerance) or, if the genes are present, celiac disease. The small intestine should be lined with what looks like pink shag carpeting. These structures are called villi and are also covered with hair-like structures called microvilli. It is through these structures that we absorb all of the nutrients from the food we eat. Healthy villi and microvilli are what provide the lock-and-key-like system that allows the good nutrients into the bloodstream, to be transported to the cells that need those nutrients to perform their duties.

The damage that occurs to the villi in celiac disease was determined and named by Dr. Michael Marsh in 1992, and the "Marsh" system of categorizing celiac damage has been the medical standard since the intestinal biopsy for celiac disease became the "gold standard" for diagnosing celiac disease (more on that later). *Marsh I* damage leads to the microvilli being destroyed. These are the microvilli that excrete the enzymes that break down the lactose sugar in milk (lactase) and sucrose (sucrase). If a person offers that they are lactose intolerant, this should be a red flag that the microvilli may be damaged. *Marsh II* and *Marsh III* damage leads to the villi being shortened, blunted, and atrophied, and the tight junctions between the villi opening up; this damage resembles Berber carpeting. *Marsh IV* damage is when the villi become flattened, and the tissue is inflamed and edematous. Picture a hot, waterlogged sponge, or red-hot, inflamed linoleum. Keep in mind that all of this destruction constitutes organ damage.

Now those food particles, which include the wheat/gliadin protein, (a long-chain amino acid that we have no enzymes as human beings to break down), yeast, bacteria, parasites, and viruses are able to get through the now "leaky" gut barrier and into the bloodstream, where they can be transported throughout the body. If you have increased permeability of your intestinal wall, then you have leaky blood vessels, leaky lungs, leaky skin, and a leaky blood–brain barrier. None of which is a good thing, of course. Your integumentary system (the organ system that protects the body from various kinds of danger) is damaged—not just in your intestines but in your whole body. Those long-chain amino acid proteins that are now in your bloodstream are capable of damaging every organ in your body, including your brain.

This is a simple explanation of how different people with celiac disease present with a myriad of signs and symptoms. Unfortunately, most of the people who have this damage are diagnosed with many things *other than* celiac disease. Most doctors, and people in general, tend to think of celiac disease as a gastrointestinal issue that "classically" presents with chronic diarrhea and weight loss. People assume that if they don't have these "classic" symptoms, then gluten is not a problem for them. This leads to their not being appropriately screened for celiac disease when they present with any of the other 300-plus symptoms noted by Cleo Libonati, RN, in *Recognizing Celiac Disease*, which was printed in 2006. This is an excellent resource book that classifies all of celiac's related disorders and diseases based on evidence-based, peer-reviewed literature.[1] If you are a practitioner who's looking for a somewhat dated but excellent resource text, *Recognizing Celiac Disease* is it. I used to tell people that unless they went to see their doctor for a hangnail, I wanted celiac disease to be on every differential diagnosis list. I no longer say that because hangnails are a sign and symptom of nutritional deficiencies.

What is also coming to light is that celiac disease presents more frequently as neurological disturbances than the typical or "classic" gastrointestinal symptoms. When I was a nurse working in emergency departments, I distinctly remember having conversations with other nurses regarding all the "frequent

1. As time has passed and more research has been completed, I am certain *Recognizing Celiac Disease* will be revised with many more related diagnoses, but it may soon become too big to lift due to all of the recent research that's being published. Regardless, you can go to http://www.glutenfreeworks.com to get the wealth of updated information.

flyers" and drug-seeking patients who came through the ED continuously. What if we had been missing a whole disease or something else that was causing all of those recurrent symptoms? We certainly weren't curing these patients of their migraines, fibromyalgia, or other pain issues with shots of Demerol and Phenergan or Toradol or Dilaudid and Zofran. They would get an injection or two and be sent home to sleep in a dark room. It was not uncommon for these patients to return after the narcotics wore off and their migraine or pain was back. We rarely, if ever, identified or effectively treated the underlying issue.

Shortly after I was almost diagnosed with celiac disease, I began to immerse myself in learning everything I possibly could about my "rare" condition. I quickly realized that it is not rare at all, but tends to be misdiagnosed as many, many different things. When I was diagnosed, by accident, with dermatitis herpetiformis and celiac disease in October 2006, my doctor thought it was rare because according to the medical textbooks, celiac disease occurred at a rate of 1 in 5,000 to 10,000. And that *would* be considered rare. But in the past few years since then, that rate has dropped to 1 in 2,500, then 1 in 1,000, then 1 in 750, 1 in 500, 1 in 350, 1 in 250, 1 in 133… and it currently sits at 1 in 100. Can you see the trend? Keep in mind that these numbers are primarily for people of European descent. White people. Most ethnic groups have not been adequately tested by any standards.

This is for those people who argue that "we have been eating wheat for ten thousand years." Unless your ancestors come from an area around the "fertile crescent" of Mesopotamia, present-day Kuwait, the northeastern part of Syria, and parts of Turkey and Iran, then "we" have *not* been eating wheat or similar grains for 10,000 years. However, if you would like to focus on that area of the world, there is plenty of scientific evidence showing that celiac disease is just as prevalent there—or even more so—than in other areas of the world.

The only World Health Organization (WHO)-funded study regarding celiac disease was completed and reported in 1999 by Dr. Carlo Catassi and his team. A study was done on Sahrawi children in Algeria showing a celiac rate of 1 in 18 in the pediatric population. I found this information fascinating and compelling. Two of the primary focus issues for the WHO are diarrheal illnesses and recognizing and decreasing the "burden of disease." I looked for more WHO-funded studies related to celiac disease in the literature and I could not find much, if anything. I eventually emailed Dr. Catassi to ask what was being done with this information and when the follow-up research was going to be reported. He very kindly emailed back that nothing was being done with this information and there were no plans for a follow-up study. This is interesting, because even just taking into account children presenting with chronic diarrhea as a primary symptom, diarrheal illnesses are supposed to be a main focus for WHO because of the high morbidity and mortality rates associated with these illnesses.

Delayed puberty, which is described as late onset of secondary and tertiary sexual development such as hair growth, breast development, initial menses or onset of first menstrual period, etc., is an indicator of potential celiac disease. These young adults are physically and hormonally primed for infertility issues and complications related to pregnancy. If a man or a woman presents to a doctor in Finland with infertility issues, the number-one thing they are tested for is celiac disease. But if these same people present to the doctor in the United States, celiac disease is not even suggested as a possibility.

The United States' medical system is set up for profit-driven health care, not for the benefit of the patient. The options presented to women and men seeking to get pregnant are typically in vitro fertilization (IVF) or some other highly expensive, technically challenging, invasive procedure. Here is what these patients *aren't* told: If you are an undiagnosed mom attempting to carry a child in your uterus full-term, but your issues of inflammation, autoimmunity, malnutrition, and leaky intestines are not corrected prior to becoming pregnant, your chances of carrying that pregnancy to term are diminished. This means your risk of miscarriage, a low-birth-weight baby, neural defects such as spina bifida, and stillbirth are increased because you have not corrected all of these issues before the pregnancy was established.

Just a few of the issues associated with babies of undiagnosed celiac moms and dads include failure to thrive, digestive issues, eczema, constipation, seizure disorders, Down, Turner, and Williams syndromes, and further down the road, a much higher rate of mental health issues such as anxiety, depression, bipolar, and schizophrenia. These kids may have learning disabilities such as dyslexia and may be diagnosed with ADD, ADHD, oppositional defiant disorder (ODD), and other learning disabilities. They may also have anger issues that don't make any sense, temper tantrums that arise out of thin air, perhaps because their brains are inflamed by the foods they are eating.

These undiagnosed children do not achieve as well as children and adults without celiac disease. They may have lower IQ scores. They have a harder time in school with focusing, learning, retaining information, and excelling. As adults, they have diminished earning power, are less likely to climb the corporate ladder, and often struggle to stay afloat in a relentless world.

All in the Family

When I found out I was pregnant at the age of twenty-one, I weighed 120 pounds and was (and still am) five foot nine and three-quarter inches tall. I was certainly malnourished then, and by all rights should not have been able to maintain a pregnancy. But somehow, intrinsically or intuitively, I knew I had to change my diet and take better care of myself. I ate more meat, fish, fruits, and vegetables, and was able to quickly put on ten pounds. I did not stop eating gluten because I didn't know any better. For this, I am forever sad. But I took being a pregnant woman very seriously. I did the best I could at the time with what little I knew.

I did successfully carry and deliver my son, Rory, shortly after my twenty-second birthday. He was a whopping eight pounds, thirteen ounces. I swore then and there that I would never birth another child. I looked around at the women who were on their second or third babies, and just didn't understand how they would decide to knowingly go through that excruciating pain more than once. My plan had been to have a natural childbirth with no pain medications. I have a super high pain tolerance—it is another one of those redhead traits. But it wasn't long after my labor started progressing that I was yelling at the nurse, like a junkie strung out and needing a fix in a bad way, to bring me my fucking Nubain and give it to me NOW. If the human species had been relying on me to replicate and populate, we would have been extinct a long time ago. To this day, just remembering the pain makes me shudder.

I was determined to breastfeed my son, which I did for eighteen months. At that time in American history, breastfeeding was not as in vogue as it is today. I loved breastfeeding, despite the initial cracked and bleeding nipples. I loved bonding with my baby and always having his food ready, warm, and what I thought was nourishing. It must have been enough, because he grew, developed, and met all of his milestones. What happened next, though, scared the ever-loving crap out of me. At the age of eighteen months, when I stopped breastfeeding, Rory developed inguinal, where his body and his leg come together, lymph nodes swelling on the right side. I took him to his pediatrician, who did an exam and drew his blood. I was unaware during the initial visit that they were working him up for non-Hodgkin's lymphoma (NHL). And I was still young and dumb enough that I didn't really know what that meant, thankfully. A biopsy of his lymph nodes was scheduled and performed. But it wasn't NHL or any other form of cancer. As a matter of fact, none of the local pathologists could diagnose whatever "it" was.

So my son's lymph tissue was sent to a pathologist out of state, who diagnosed atypical mycobacterium avium intercellulare, which is not uncommon in late-stage HIV patients. Hmmmm. My son was not infected with HIV. We didn't own birds. We weren't even much for bird watching other than out our windows at home. To this day, this diagnosis makes no sense whatsoever. Thankfully, there has been no reoccurrence.

But what ended happily and unremarkably seemed to also trigger my super-funny and sweet son into a fairly consistent state of the terrible twos, which lasted until he was eighteen years old. The first memorable event occurred around Christmas time. My cousin, Tracy, and I were at a mall with Rory shopping for gifts. As we walked into the first store from the parking lot, Rory started to headbutt me, and not lightly. Once the tantrums began, it was hard to get a handle on his behavior. He seemed so angry, but we certainly couldn't figure out what our two-year-old had to be angry about—especially one who was extremely well loved and tended to by a broad community of family and friends, and who was eating the standard American diet of Cheerios, orange fish, and plenty of fruits and vegetables.

As Rory got older and started preschool, kindergarten and first grade, it became clear we had our hands full. We would get reports of his being very smart, and he tested into the talented and gifted program, but his behavior was abysmal. At his first grade parent–teacher conference attended by his dad and myself, we were excited to hear good things and what Rory was learning. His first grade teacher, however, declared, out loud, that my son was a "devil child." I had seen Damian in *Omen* 1, 2, and 3, and I knew what that meant. Whoa. Of course, the Momma Bear kicked in and I voiced my opinion of her abilities as a first grade teacher, and then reported that Rory would not be back to her classroom after winter break, and he wasn't.

Rory's next first grade class was a first and second grade split. His new teacher had over twenty-five years' experience teaching children. Despite all of her vast experience and understanding, though, Rory now had a desk outside of the principal's office with his name on it. We had numerous meetings with the school's teachers and principals for disciplinary actions and possible testing options. Rory fought us constantly, over homework, food, bedtime, or whatever else was making him angry at that moment.

Rory and I went on a three-week driving trip around the East Coast when he was just starting first grade. We started in Buffalo, then drove to D.C. to stay with friends and see the sights. Jacqueline "Jackie" Kennedy had recently died, so we visited her grave site at Arlington Cemetery. I explained the eternal flame to Rory. I told him, "It will never go out. That's why it is called the eternal flame." He immediately disagreed with me, and for the rest of the trip this became the topic of discussions and disagreements. We laugh about it now, but at the time, when he was six years old, he was wearing my patience thin.

We saw pediatricians, psychologists, and psychiatrists. We saw counselors and more counselors. I made a point of asking every one of these people if there was any chance my son's behavior was being negatively influenced by the foods I was feeding him. Unequivocally, I was told his behavior had nothing to do with the food he was eating. I was advised to medicate him, which never happened because I would not let him be medicated. His pediatrician also told me my job, as his mother, was to keep him out of prison. Wow.

Rory's teenage years brought more than our fair share of challenges. While he could be the sweetest kid in the world, there were many times he pushed everyone's limits, above and well beyond any acceptable range. My deepest regret and enormous guilt as a mother stems from not knowing I was a celiac or even a gene carrier before I got pregnant. I absolutely, without a doubt, would have gone gluten free at the very least, for the health and development of my baby. I think of all of that wasted time, energy, and money spent chasing something that would have helped my son and our family, and it makes me sad and angry. I asked all of the right questions. But I never did get the right answer for myself, or for my son before he was nineteen years old and well on his way to becoming a responsible adult.

Even though we have determined Rory is an HLA-DQ2.5 gene carrier and a homozygous gene carrier for gluten-sensitivity genes, he remains on a gluten-containing diet. Rory assures me that he will gladly go on a gluten free diet, but not until after he tests positive for celiac disease. However, my grandpuppy, Harlow, is on a grain-free diet. My grandpuppy is Paleo! There is hope for my son and my future grandchildren yet.

Celiac disease is genetic. It gets passed down from generation to generation. Each subsequent generation becomes sicker, and it takes them longer to heal. It can take several generations to undo the damage that has been done. Both of my parents were gene carriers for DQ2.5. That would have been a good thing for my parents to know before they started popping out kids, as good Catholics were known to do in the '50s and '60s. My mother had at least two miscarriages that she knows of, and the twin boys, Michael and Matthew, who were born two years before me, were born prematurely and died shortly after birth. My mother gave birth to five children who lived; I was number four in 1966. I can say with a fair amount of certainty that I had celiac disease while in utero.

Of course, I didn't learn this priceless nugget of information until I was forty years old and almost dead. But being a good person in general, and a nurse, I didn't think it a wise idea to keep this knowledge to myself. So I told everyone my story and what I was learning. More than one person in my life has advised me to "temper my enthusiasm," but here I am, eight years later, and still enthusiastic. I called up my siblings and told them they had to get tested whether they had symptoms or not. They also needed to get my nieces and nephews tested for celiac disease. I knew their medical histories.

I also know that we are a trophy-winning family capable of

burping and farting like you can't imagine. In high school, I was gifted with a fart jar for one of my birthdays. Some kids had collections of fancy dolls or trinkets. I collected fart and burp paraphernalia and books. I am surprised my friends are still my friends after breaking wind in their presence so many times and with little or no grace. Farting was always funny, up to a point. Usually until someone was thrown into an asthma attack and had to use their emergency inhaler. We produced enough methane gas as a family to have significantly contributed to global warming. I apologize to the world for this contribution. I just didn't know it wasn't the beans. My dad, with his funky polio gait, would walk across the kitchen floor, fart, and then state, "The floor boards must be loose again." Or, "Someone must have let the ducks out." My grandmother, my dad's mother, would claim she was "shooting the guy behind me." Like I said, we were champions, and we embraced our familial talent to produce gas with gusto.

So I've suspected that everyone in my family has celiac disease, and I know we are all, on both sides of my family, genetically predisposed to celiac disease. None of this is quantum physics. It all makes sense. But sadly, it is the common-sense part that is often lacking, when denial sets in like a ten-ton dinosaur and causes an extreme refusal to believe anything outside the box of the "known" comfort zone. A year and a half after I kindly informed my family that I have celiac disease and told them to get tested, my sister, three years younger than I, called me up to tell me my nine-year-old niece was in the hospital. Why was my nine-year old niece in the hospital, I asked, concerned. My sister explained that the pediatric surgeon was prepping to take my niece's gallbladder and spleen out because she had genetic spherocytosis, which causes anemia and an enlarged spleen. WHAT?!? We don't even take out spleens that are traumatically injured. They get meshed and left in place. Spleens are important in ways we don't even understand yet, and they are a phenomenally important part of the immune system. Who takes out a nine-year-old's gallbladder and spleen?!?

I anxiously asked if they had actually tested her for celiac disease and was informed that no, they hadn't. So I said, "Have them test her for celiac. That's what she has. Tell the pediatric surgeon to put his scalpel down and have him order a celiac panel. She has celiac disease," I said confidently. "Change her diet and she will get better. Whatever she has, is caused by eating gluten. Get her tested, now, before she has her gallbladder and spleen removed, for Christ's sake!"

I hung up the phone with my sister, and three hours later, she called back. "Surgery was a success," she said. "They took out her gallbladder and spleen." (Holy Mother of Mary, pray for us.)

My mother has always been "unpleasant." As far as I know, that has always been the case. As a matter of fact, I moved out of her house when I was thirteen years old. The day I graduated from eighth grade, I was packed up and my dad picked me up right after school. I was waiting by the back door with my few boxes of kid treasures. I moved into my dad's brand-new third wife Marie's house—out of the frying pan and into the fire.

My dad, Phil, was always kind and just a nice, nice man. He had "sucker" written all over his face. Even though he was a salesman of industrial equipment, he really could be sold anything. He was a pretty simple guy. Unfortunately, he was also stricken with the poliovirus as a toddler. His left leg was severely atrophied and devoid of muscle. My dad endured multiple surgeries as a child and as an adult. He refused to allow the doctors to amputate his almost useless left leg. It was significantly shorter than his right, normal leg. He had to wear two different-sized shoes and then had to have significant lifts added to the left one. He wore a brace on his left leg at all times because his knee would just collapse. But my dad was not a complainer or a whiner or a victim. He just was who he was. Polio stopped him from roller skating, running, and skiing, but he managed to do almost everything else and he certainly made it possible for us to take part in all of the activities he was physically unable to do.

My daughter Hannah and I visited my dad last summer. Hannah very much wanted to see her Grandpa Phil after he had been diagnosed with bone cancer and put in hospice care because, as she said, "My grandpa always loved me, always." Hannah was a newborn when she became our daughter via adoption, and my dad flew immediately out to Oregon to meet her. He quite obviously adored her at first sight.

When we first arrived at the facility, we were directed to a room down a long hallway. As Hannah and I headed in the direction of my dad's room, a caregiver was pushing a man in a wheelchair toward us. My initial impression was, "Oh! There's my dad!" But as we got closer, I was less sure that this man was my dad. He sort of looked like my dad. This man was really bloated and somehow didn't look like my dad. I looked at Hannah and she looked and me and we both shrugged. Neither of us was sure.

It wasn't until we were almost past this man that I spoke. "Dad?"

His watery-blue eyes looked at me with a sudden sparkle and said, "I didn't know you were coming! I am so happy you are here. Look at my girl Hannah! You are so beautiful!"

Each day we would visit, he had forgotten the previous day. Which was fine with us, because then he got to be excited and happy all over again, each day. During that visit, I requested that my dad be tested for celiac disease. I spoke to one of the RNs on shift who knew my dad well. I explained that I was a gene carrier for celiac disease, that I have celiac disease, and I know my dad gave me one of the two DQ2.5 genes I carry. I explained that I am an expert in celiac disease and gluten intolerance. I gave her my Gluten Free RN business card and asked her to please have the doctor call me if there were any questions. I eventually did hear through the family grapevine that one of the nurses from the facility called my brother and said the doctor refused to order the celiac disease panel. Ouch. The reasons given were that he was old and there was no way they could or would feed him a gluten-free diet, even if he had celiac disease.

This past February, before my dad died in May, Rory and I visited him in the skilled nursing facility where he was housed. His memory certainly wasn't getting better, but he struggled valiantly to remember Polish words and stories from the past. I was particularly interested in the Polish swear words my grandma, "Doc," would verbalize when she was less than happy about something. We had really great visits with him each day. Rory, a paramedic/firefighter, had spent the previous summer employed at Yellowstone National Park in the Old Faithful District. He showed his grandpa amazing photos and told him stories about his work, the bison, the geysers, and everything about his summer. I took photos of Rory's and my dad's hands together. I also took a cheek swab for a DNA test for celiac disease from my dad. I explained to my dad what I was doing, why, and my theories of why his dad, who was a baker, had died at the young age of sixty from kidney failure.

I am forever thankful for these last visits my kids and I had with my dad. During the same trip, my niece celebrated her sixteenth birthday. What does a loving Aunt Nini get her beloved niece for her sixteenth birthday? A DNA test for celiac disease, of course! A few weeks later, the genetic test results for my dad and my niece arrived via email. My dad's results showed him to be homozygous for HLA-DQ2.5. Which means he was bequeathed genes for celiac disease from his mother and father. He was pretty much guaranteed to have celiac disease, but was never tested and certainly not diagnosed. Another Super Celiac. And my niece? What did her test show? She is also homozygous for HLA-DQ2.5. She received genes from her mother, my sister, and her father. Another Super Celiac. If you remember, this is the niece who had her gallbladder and spleen removed when she was nine years old. Damage done.

Gluten Free – and Just the Beginning

A few days after my initial blood draw and skin biopsy for celiac disease and dermatitis in Dr. Haberman's office, we set off on a planned family trip to New York City. In researching celiac disease, I had discovered there was a celiac disease center at Columbia University and that the center would be hosting an International Celiac Disease Symposium while we were there on vacation. I thought long and hard about attending the symposium, but in the end, fun time with my family won out.

I did the best I could to maintain a gluten-free diet in New York City during that trip. I was also very, very sad because at my favorite places to eat, such as Carmine's Italian Restaurant, I could only have salad with no croutons, the best part of the salad. They were so good, in fact, that Brad and I had always ordered a side of extra croutons! No more croutons, not for me. When I traveled, my primary goal had always been to find the best bakeries and in New York City, that meant bagels (plural) with cream cheese and lox, pastries, and soft-on-the-inside, crusty-on-the-outside bread to dip into olive oil and balsamic vinegar. I loved my gluten, but clearly my gluten was not interested in our love affair anymore. Gluten had turned my love, affection, and complete devotion into some malicious monster that had been triggered into actively trying to kill me.

When we returned home, I called up Dr. Haberman's office and asked for Nurse Helen. "Hi, Nurse Helen," I said. "I am calling for my test results."

At this point, I was feeling confident that Dr. Haberman had discovered my rare disease and I was going to live and the testing was going to confirm the diagnosis. Try to imagine my complete and utter deflation when she informed me that my blood test for celiac disease was negative and the skin biopsy showed lichen planus, not dermatitis herpetiformis. Nurse Helen said I had a rash because I scratched my skin.

I was dumbfounded and devastated. My tests were negative. The negative tests pretty much confirmed what had been insinuated by the multitude of doctors I had seen. I WAS, in fact, crazy. I HAD made up all of my symptoms, including my 4+ pitting edema and my swollen and painful lymph nodes. I was CAUSING the rash that was pure and unadulterated torture day and night. Out of the last vestiges of my very essence came a primal, guttural cry of resignation. I was going to die. Fine. Good. Let me die.

Brad and our kids received the news, digested it, and said, "Wow, Mom, you *are* crazy!" They laughed, but then said, "Hey, look, you're clearly better on this stupid diet. We can see the difference. You're getting better. Why don't you just stay on it and see what happens?"

At this point, I clearly had nothing to lose by staying on this stupid gluten-free diet, and I WAS undeniably feeling better. So I did.

When I went back to see Dr. Haberman for a follow-up appointment, I said, "I didn't listen to you. I started getting better almost immediately on a diet without gluten, so despite my negative tests, I stayed on it, and I am getting better!

She hung her head, looked at the floor, and said, "Scientifically, it doesn't make any sense; your tests were negative. You should not be getting better."

I gleefully said, "Yes, but I am."

"Yes, I see that," she said.

The next time I saw Dr. Haberman, she herself was on a gluten-free, dairy-free, soy-free diet. She called me a few months later and said, "Don't eat corn either." Dr. Haberman changed the way she practices medicine and dermatology because she realized that had I listened to her, I would have most assuredly been dead. That's one of the benefits of being a nurse. We don't always listen to doctors. But when nurses and doctors collaborate, magic happens.

When I was still at a loss as to what health-care provider to reach out to who could possibly help me get better, I called around to a few alternative practitioners' offices and rather crankily asked if they had ever worked with someone who couldn't eat gluten?

To my surprise, Dr. Leslie Berman's receptionist replied affirmatively: "Of course Dr. Berman can help you! She is gluten free too. She is really great."

I thought she sounded either exceptionally delusional or really optimistic. Did she really think there were other people who would be on a gluten-free diet or who understood my really rare disease and could actually help me?

Dr. Berman, a chiropractor, essentially did nutritional critical care for me. Helped me heal my intestines. Brain fog gone. Suddenly, the sky was much bluer than it had ever been before. She put me on an elimination diet, which my 10-year-old daughter, Hannah, did with me. Hannah said she felt better within 24 hours of going gluten free. My muscles were still like rocks; I saw massage therapists, chiropractors, acupuncturists and every "alternative" practitioner I could to help my body heal. My doctors argued with me; I fired them at a record pace, and sometimes they fired me first. I even requested a heavy metal test because of a persistent metallic taste in my mouth. My urine test came back high positive for arsenic. I had to ask my husband, Brad, if those gluten-free donuts he was feeding me were laced with arsenic. We laughed about it, but I was still suspicious because after I asked him, those symptoms went away… I honestly don't think he was poisoning me.

Within four months, I felt so much better that I took pencil to tri-folded paper and designed the brochure for my new company, RN On Call, Inc. I had never thought about being an entrepreneur before, but suddenly I had the energy, brainpower, and total ignorance of what it takes to start up and run a business, like I had never experienced before. Somehow, I found out about an organization called NNBA, National Nurses in Business, run by an emergency nurse named Pat Bemis. Pat spent quality hours on the phone with me, patiently answering all of my questions and advising me about everything I would need to be successful.

RN On Call, Inc. is a melding of in-home nursing visits, which include all doctor-ordered procedures, lab draws, vital signs, and exams, management of health-care appointments and end-of-life care. Many of my clients have no family, or family that lives in another state or another country. I am an advocate for them as they navigate the aging process, typically in-home, and make sure they are aware of options available to them as their situation changes. My clients pay me directly, and I work for them to make sure their wishes are followed.

As an example, one of my dear clients had been in the hospital five to six times every year with pneumonia and long rehabilitation periods following each hospitalization. After she became my client, she was able to stay out of the hospital and in her own home for the remaining three years she was alive. Her quality of life was much improved. If there was any indicator of infection or medical problems, I was called, assessed her situation, and reviewed her options for care and treatment with her and her primary care provider. There were periods of time I saw her once a week and other times once or more a day. It was important to her to have an advocate and a professional who would help be her voice. She died peacefully in her own bed, as she had wished, surrounded by people who loved her.

Over the past eight years, I have been blessed with some wonderful people to work with and for as their private nurse. This is another part of my work that is individualized for each client. Some of my favorite clients have been a challenge—what some people would call "grumpy" or hard to get along with. For this reason, and for many more, all of my RN On Call clients get tested for celiac disease every year. The best part of working with them and their families is that I do not have the issues with the mom or the dad that the adult children sometimes have—although I certainly understand and respect what some of those issues may involve. I am not a nurse bully with my lovely clients, and I want them to be as healthy, happy, and active as possible for their remaining time, whether it is a few months or many years.

This is the business model that allowed me to financially support my work as the Gluten Free RN once I stopped working as an agency nurse in emergency departments in December 2007. If I had simply stayed in the RN On Call business and continued to pull a salary from my work, I would have been set and making a decent living. But by financially supporting what some people initially called my gluten-free educational "hobby" as the Gluten Free RN, my bank accounts are not always overflowing with profits. After I started working in the emergency department in 1993, I would declare to myself, my family, and my friends that I was so elated to be an emergency/trauma nurse that I would have paid to do it! Well, here I find myself seventeen years later doing that exact thing, paying to do work I love and that I feel compelled to provide.

After starting RN On Call, I continued to work my agency shifts, full-time plus overtime shifts in emergency departments, all over the state of Oregon. I never took a sick day, and I never missed a beat. The same Polish tenacity and bullheadedness that had kept me going despite multi-system organ failure was now kicking in, and I was feeling truly alive for the first time in years. I had meetings with attorneys, bookkeepers, accountants, and printers. I was way, way far out of my comfort zone but surprisingly undeterred. During this same time of eating gluten free and healing, I researched and read voraciously about gluten and celiac disease. I read everything I could get my hands on from the library, the Internet, and celiac organizations.

I also called Alice Bast from the National Foundation for Celiac Awareness. We had a terrific/terrifying conversation regarding her story of multiple miscarriages and stillbirths before a diagnosis of celiac disease. From my perspective as a former New Yorker, I asked her if she was ever afraid of "swimming with the fishes" because she was potentially threatening to the food and wheat industries. She told me that this was a concern her friends and family had mentioned, but that she was unflappable in her resolve to speak out about celiac disease.

The first book I got my hands on about celiac disease was written by Peter Green, MD, and Rory Jones from the Celiac Disease Center at Columbia University entitled *Celiac Disease: A Hidden Epidemic.* I read it and reread it. I made my nurse friends read it. I bought extra copies and gave it to people. I frequently took it to work with me in the ED. I started asking patients at triage if they had ever been tested for celiac. I also started to reevaluate our "frequent flyers" and drug-seeking patients for celiac. Most of the patients I would ask about being tested for celiac said things like, "My doctors think I am crazy." "My doctors put me on all of these meds but they don't help." "I am only twenty-one years old, but I am just exhausted all of the time and I can't think."

One of the patient interactions that stands out for me as a nurse occurred during this period. A lady had presented to the ED with a rash that covered her face and most of her body. It was extremely painful and extremely itchy. The only thing that would make it feel better was sitting naked in front of a fan. The air would relieve some of the pain and itching. I looked at the rash and immediately told the doctor on duty that day that I knew what that rash was! It was dermatitis herpetiformis, and this nice lady had celiac disease. I requested he order the celiac panel that was mentioned in the book on celiac disease and written by a DOCTOR, an actual MD.

This particular ED doctor, however, had a reputation of being sexist, grumpy, resentful, and not easy to work with. I could elaborate, but you get the idea. I showed him the reference to the test. I found the lab test in the computer. At first he refused, vehemently, but I can be tenacious and persuasive and unrelenting. He finally, reluctantly gave in, and I drew the blood and sent it to the lab, knowing the lab was a send-out and the results wouldn't be back for two or three days. I printed up the discharge instructions, which basically said, "You have a rash and we do not know what it is or what causes it." The doctor had also written out two prescriptions for prednisone and triamcinolone cream.

I sat down on the swirly stool at her bedside, handed her the discharge sheet, and said, "We don't know what is causing your rash, but the doctor agreed to run a celiac blood panel test."

She said, "Is that when you can't eat gluten?"

I looked at her crosswise and said, "Yes. How do you know that it is related to gluten?"

She replied, "Because all my grandchildren are on a gluten-free diet. My daughter knows all about it. Some of her kids were sick and once they stopped eating gluten, they got better!"

I laughed and said, "Well, since it's genetic, they probably got it from you!"

We both took a deep breath and laughed. Then, based on the information in the book stating that prednisone is contraindicated for celiac patients and that the triamcinolone cream wouldn't help with dermatitis herpetiformis, after talking about it with the patient, I ripped up the prescriptions and gave them back to the doc. He looked at the ripped prescriptions, and then he looked at me and tossed them into the recycling box.

After that, all of my patients who came to the emergency department, regardless of what they came in for, were given at least one dose of prednisone by this particular doctor. Harmful to patients that didn't need prednisone? Malpractice? Ouch.

It was also during one of these shifts in the emergency department that the unit secretary informed me I had a phone call from New York. Typically, no one called me at work because I was busy, sometimes working hard to save a life or two or seven. Certainly, no one from New York would call me at work unless it was urgent. I barely spoke to any of my family members who lived in Buffalo in general, and certainly not while I was at work. With the expectation that someone on the other end of that phone call was going to tell me one of my parents had died, I picked up the phone. On the end was my younger sister, Lori.

"Hey, what's up?" I said.

"Ian's dead," she said.

Stunned.

Ian was my big, brown-eyed, nineteen-year-old nephew who was six months older than my own son, Rory. Those boys had played together fabulously, and Ian had spent some of his summer vacations having adventures with us in Oregon.

My nurse friends started to pay attention to my conversation as the tone of my voice changed and I began asking all of the questions that come to one's mind when faced with an unexpected death of a young loved one. When? What happened? Was he in a car accident? The story at this point, what I could gather from my sister, was that Ian's older brother, my nephew Collin, had found him dead in his bed. I hadn't seen Ian in a few years. I recalled that he had had issues with drug abuse, but that he had gone through a rehab program and was doing great.

The unremarkable fact was that he had drug abuse issues, because especially if you were a male in our family, drug and alcohol addictions ran long and deep throughout our family history. Most of the men lived brutally hard, unpleasant lives, abused their wives and children, and then died young of things like cirrhosis of the liver or flying cars that took down three telephone poles and ejected the unbelted occupants, both of whom I was related to. One died, my cousin Wayne, and one lived, my brother Greg. Ian was Greg's son, and now he was dead too.

So begins this particular saga of epic proportions.

On to Something

In February 2007, I had just received the first printing of my shiny brochures for RN On Call, Inc. My business! But before I could do anything with those brochures or announce to the world that I was open for business, the call came about Ian's death. I packed up a few of the brochures to show my friends and family, and Rory and I made the journey back to Buffalo, New York, for Ian's funeral.

We arrived in Buffalo with only a few hours to spare before my nephew was to be cremated. Because we had minimal notice, I hadn't arranged for a rental car. One of my best friends from high school picked us up at the airport and the plan was to get a rental car the next morning. The bad news was, there were no rental cars to be had in Buffalo that day, for some unexplainable reason. I called and called and called rental car companies and car dealerships without any luck, getting more and more frustrated and feeling thwarted in my effort to view my nephew's body.

Finally, in a fit of despair, I relayed to some poor man on the other end of the line that if I did not get a rental car soon, we would not get to view my nineteen-year-old nephew's body before he was cremated. There was silence on the other end of the line. I was put on hold, and when the man came back, he asked where they could deliver a car, in about fifteen minutes. True to the man's word, a car driven by a sweet young man was delivered to us in less than fifteen minutes.

Rory and I made it to the funeral home in time. Ian was in the front viewing room, on a stretcher, zipped up in a body bag. The funeral director unzipped the bag to reveal the fabulously handsome face of my now dead and lifeless Ian. I could no longer see his big brown eyes, as they had been sealed shut. I could see the beginnings of the sewn-up chest incision that was created during his autopsy. My son and I did what grieving and family members do in the face of sudden and inexplicable death. We talked to Ian. We talked to each other. We said goodbye the best we could. What a struggle. Rory was only eighteen years old. What a horrible experience for a young adult. His cousin, his friend, his buddy, dead.

We got through the funeral and the family gatherings intact but depleted to the core. The level of dysfunction in my family runs long and deep and is certainly multi-generational. Any family gathering is typically fraught with angst and trepidation, with adrenaline surges ready at any warning sign of conflict. Fight. Run. Flee. There were no rules of etiquette for family gatherings, especially where alcohol was being consumed. And if my family was involved, alcohol, at the very least, was being consumed.

Ian's memorial service was held at a tavern in a little town south of Buffalo where the preferred mode of transportation was snowmobile. Nice. My friend Beth, fully in the know of potential conflict and said angst, drove Rory and me to the service and the after-"party." She was uniquely qualified to accompany us since she had met most, but not all of the players, my family, but also because she was intrinsically curious about how this would all play out. She knew about the potential for chaos. Remarkably, the day for us ended uneventfully with, as far as I know, everyone behaving with a modicum of respect and dignity.

After returning safely home with Rory to Corvallis, I started thinking. Was it possible that Ian had celiac too? Was it possible that all of the families' addiction issues were related to gluten? Were we all celiac? I had learned that this was genetic, but what did that mean? After giving it some thought, I came to the conclusion that I wished I had known this before Ian had died, certainly, but I would have at least requested that Ian be tested for celiac on autopsy. Since that was no longer an option, what were my options to investigate this theory?

My idea was that people with addiction issues are all potentially celiac or gluten intolerant, and I needed to test someone. I asked a young family friend, slightly older than Rory, who struggled with addiction issues to be genetically tested for celiac disease, because if my assumptions were correct, this could be a link to potentially all addiction issues. He agreed, and met me at his place of employment during off hours. He swabbed his cheek and I paid for the test.

I was shocked and excited in an odd way when his genetic test came back homozygous for HLA-DQ2. Was I on to something? Surely he would agree to get tested for the antibodies and his family would be ecstatic to learn there was hope for him and for them. I met him again, explained what I understood at the time about what the results meant, and encouraged him to get further testing. I then stopped by the house of his parents, who were best friends with my husband, and explained as best as I knew how at the time that the whole family was at risk for celiac and that their son's addiction issues quite possibly stemmed from being gluten intolerant or celiac. I was expecting a conversation. I was also expecting to explain more about how to go about testing the whole family.

Instead, the father's response was, "I can't think of anyone in my whole family that doesn't have an addiction issue. This is just something we all have." And I later learned that his son had taken to telling people that he was an addict *because* he was "celiac." Like it was his excuse for using drugs and he had no choice but to be addicted. Wow. The addiction issues are not the only sign or symptom of celiac for this family. I love them to pieces, but seriously?

As a nurse, and a triage nurse especially, it is not hard to find people who have gluten intolerance or celiac disease. It just is not hard. This is not rocket science. Plus, it is harder to find people who *don't* have gluten intolerance or celiac disease, or don't have it yet. Nurses have this ability to look at people and really see illness and impending death. That is what we should be good at, especially if we are going to sit in that emergency department window and decide who is sick enough to get taken back to a room, stat, and who to tell to sit down and wait to be called in the order we decide based on their symptoms or lack thereof. This is an extremely important skill. It always reflects poorly on the nurse who leaves a critically ill person in the waiting room when they should have been triaged as a "Type 1" or a "Type 2" who's TTD ("trying to die"). Unfortunately, this does happen, and not always with a happy ending.

As a triage nurse who has spent countless hours triaging people who present to the emergency department and immersing myself in celiac disease education, I see celiac disease, and I see it everywhere: in airports, outside my office window, in hospitals, on city streets, at conferences, and, well, everywhere. Sometimes, I think about telling people. Stopping them or calling after them just to suggest they get tested for celiac disease because they have a rash, "acne," vitiligo, facial tics or tremors, a funny gait, or some other telltale sign that makes my bells go off. DING! DING! DING! But, that would be weird. I would probably get arrested. Probably get reported and accused of harassment. Not everyone wants to be approached and told they may have a disease by a stranger in an airport, nurse or not.

But I cannot explain how much I would have appreciated someone, anyone suggesting I had an issue with my food, and that gluten and dairy could have been causing all of my medical issues. It was pure torture, being a nurse, a really good nurse, and not being able to self-diagnose, discover, or even get help in discovering that it was really my food that was killing me. Torture. The reality is my pediatricians, even as a child, or any of my doctors could have seen my celiac disease in my family, had they been looking. All of the signs were there. Many, many blaring signs and symptoms were there.

I started RN On Call in February 2007, four months after my "diagnosis by accident." By March 2007, I was so horrified by what I had found out about gluten intolerance and celiac disease that I started Gluten Free RN. My initial intent with Gluten Free RN was to educate my health-care provider friends—my people, my people who had misdiagnosed me. It took me quite a bit of time to realize my nurse and doctor friends were not interested in learning about celiac disease. How could this be?

What I came to understand is that we live in a for-profit health-care system: a system that profits from sick people. Celiac disease requires only a diet change and people tend to get better. There is no pill. There is no surgery. Just a lifelong dietary shift that somewhat miraculously fixes all types of physical and mental maladies. In Italy, it takes two to three weeks to get a proper diagnosis of celiac disease. In the United States of America, on average it takes *nine to fifteen years* to get a proper diagnosis, if ever. I am certain many people die without ever knowing it was undiagnosed celiac disease that really killed them.

When working in the EDs, I actively started to ask people at triage with long lists of diagnoses and medications whether they had ever been tested for celiac disease. Overwhelmingly, the response would be, "What's that?" Sadly, many of these patients were young or belonged to our "frequent flier club" because they came to the emergency department so often. Many of them would admit that their doctor had told them they were making up their symptoms or were just crazy. Most had been referred to mental health services. No wonder mental health services are so overwhelmed! I suggested to many of these patients that they get tested for celiac disease when they saw their primary care provider. Most of them returned to tell me their doctors refused to test them.

In December of 2007, I worked my last shift as an ED nurse. That night, a patient presented to the ED, and was placed in a room. The ED doc went in to see the patient, then came out and said, "He doesn't want to see me. He just wants to see Nurse Nadine. You have to stop doing this. We don't know how to bill for it."

Certainly, my health-care provider, my co-workers, and these patients would be happy to know that celiac *is* real, and that it was simply not being looked for or diagnosed. And it would make our jobs a whole lot easier if we were actually diagnosing and treating all of these people correctly. It's a no-brainer. People would be beating down my door to hear the good news that we'd found the answer, or at least a piece of the answer, to so many of our health problems. Not so much. Not at all. Nope. Not happening.

So this is my plea to nurses. If you work in emergency medicine and you experience patients who are "frequent flyers," narcotic drug seekers, and/or just a general pain in your ass because you see them in the ED more than you see your own friends and family: test them for celiac disease. You may feel that celiac disease is not an "emergency" test, but if you have the opportunity to figure out the underlying cause of these people's pain, drug addiction, and manipulative behavior, you have an obligation to test them. No excuses. None.

I am not a Pollyanna, fluff-and-tuck nurse. My job in the ED was to quickly recognize a sick person and act accordingly. There were a few times in my career when I failed to appreciate a patient's tanking situation. These events do not make me proud of myself, but thankfully, another nurse or ED doc stepped up and pointed out what I was missing. Those are always humbling experiences that are burned into my brain to help me avoid repeating the same error in judgment or assessment.

For all of my ED doctor and nurse colleagues, trust me, I understand our roles as emergency medical personnel as far as recognizing sick people and acting appropriately. Are you in danger of dying? No. Great. Go home and follow up with your primary doctor. Unfortunately for us and for our patients, emergency departments have become the only place for many people to acquire any medical attention. The reality is, we saw, and you still see, a ton of people with mental health issues, failure to cope, and a lack of appropriate medical resources or social support. It would be great if we could triage people effectively and have them be seen at appropriate health-care venues rather than clogging up our waiting rooms and emergency departments, so that we could see only see the sick, true emergency patients: the gory traumas, heart attacks, strokes, seizures, and wounds. That's what I signed up for when I was a young nurse.

Our duty as nurses, all nurses, working in every capacity, is to protect the patient, sometimes from other nurses or doctors, to speak up for vulnerable patients, whoever they may be or how they present, and to do no harm. To the latter I would say, don't be unwarrantedly punitive to combative patients—for instance, by putting in a 14-gauge IV when an 18-gauge will do, and stay alert and up to date with current literature and research. Change is happening every second, whether it is with standards of care or new equipment, and these changes may or may not be beneficial to patient care.

So, nurses, ask yourself, "What do I know about gluten intolerance and celiac disease?" If your answer is "nothing," then you have some work to do. Considering that celiac disease is the number one autoimmune disease in the world, and you as a nurse are not looking for it in 2015, then we need to talk.

Several years ago, I gave a lecture to nursing students at our local community college. The nursing professor, also celiac, had noted that there were no chapters on celiac disease in the nursing curriculum, even in the gastrointestinal section, nor were there any NCLEX test questions. “Why are we not teaching about celiac disease in nursing school? How do we change this?” she asked.

Nurses are in a unique position to recognize signs and symptoms, and to request testing and follow-up for patients, especially ones who are critically ill. It is not uncommon for me to see patients who have a new diagnosis of celiac disease recently discharged from the ICU. They were tested for “everything” until the test for celiac disease was finally run, and lo and behold, that’s what was causing them to end up in the ICU. Medical practitioners in other countries may be dumbstruck and even horrified to learn, however, that these patients are still discharged without a follow-up plan, required baseline labs are not ordered, and if a patient is referred to a nutritionist or to someone like me, insurance companies in the United States do not pay for the appointment, even though the treatment for celiac disease is a 100 percent lifelong gluten-free diet. The treatment is merely a diet change, but these people have to pay out of pocket to see the few qualified practitioners who can actually help them. This is a barrier to care that is unbelievable, but true.

After I read *Celiac Disease: the Hidden Epidemic* by Peter Green, MD, I had everyone who expressed an interest read it. Some other nurses began wondering if this was the cause of their own symptoms. Most others, though, were tougher nuts to crack. But why? Why would they not accept the fact that we had simply failed to diagnose a major disease for well over sixty years? One of the ED docs I worked with has four kids, two of whom had been diagnosed somewhere on the autism spectrum. He and his wife spent countless hours advocating for their kids in the school system. Both kids were on Individual Education Plans, and the parents frequently had to do battle with the school districts to provide services to these kids. I suggested to him that the kids get tested for celiac. I also offered to come and help his family get started on a gluten-free diet. To this he said that he didn't want to inconvenience the rest of the family—while he was eating wheat crackers! This seemed so simple, such the obvious answer. I could not understand how anyone could NOT see it, plain as day.

What he very kindly, condescendingly said to me was, "I don't need you to tell me anything about celiac disease, thank you. I already know all about it."

I said excitedly, "You do? How do you know about it?"

"My wife's sister has celiac disease, so we are checked out on it."

Oh. Really. If your wife's sister has celiac, your wife is most likely a gene carrier, if not celiac too, and therefore, so are your children. Duh. But despite my best arguments, and presenting him with the latest research linking learning disabilities with gluten, he dismissed my concerns point-blank. I have since heard through the grapevine that he and his whole family are now on a gluten-free diet. I sure hope that's true, for the kids' sake. And I sure hope he no longer feels inconvenienced.

When I began researching, I truly believed I had a rare disease, but several events quickly and irrefutably changed my mind. I experienced what some would call a paradigm shift. Everything I learned started to build, and I realized with perfect clarity that celiac disease IS everywhere. It is huge. Enormous. I purchased Cleo Libonati's book, *Recognizing Celiac Disease,* which links celiac disease with over 300 signs and symptoms. At this point, I shifted into being much more of a public health nurse. If my colleagues were not going to listen, I would take the information to the people.

I started giving classes on what I'd learned. I had a logo made for Gluten Free RN. I had it trademarked. I made another brochure and had a thousand printed. I set up a booth at the local farmers market. I went to women's festivals. I made a tri-fold display with symptoms. I took my booth and all of my information on the road. I talked to people every day about celiac disease.

At one of the Corvallis Farmers' Market days, I had my table set up and was eagerly greeting friends and new people. Two people approached whom I recognized as an emergency room doctor and one of the emergency nurses from a coastal hospital.

The doc asked me, "What are you doing this for?" in her Scottish brogue. She is of short stature, addicted to artisan bread, with a short temper and high blood pressure.

I explained what I was doing and why.

"Celiac disease is common in Europe," she said. "I have often thought that I have celiac disease, but it doesn't exist here in the United States."

I looked at her dumbfounded. Did she think the genes got scrubbed off when we crossed the ocean? This was a bright, seemingly well-educated woman making a statement that made absolutely no sense whatsoever. My highly educated guess is that yes, she is correct, and she too is celiac.

As I started to look around and become more aware of how celiac actually presented, I began to have a super-high index of suspicion for just about everyone. In the fall of 2007, events continued to occur that cemented my resolve to focus on celiac disease. One such event was when I heard Dr. Jerome Groopman being interviewed on NPR for his book *How Doctors Think*. In the interview, Dr. Groopman told the tale of a woman who was misdiagnosed for years with anorexia and bulimia, put in mental institutions, accused of lying and making up her symptoms, and so on. One exceptional doctor finally saw her, listened to her story, and talked her into getting a test for celiac, which is what she ended up being diagnosed with. All those years of being misdiagnosed, mistreated, and charged for it, and come to find out all of those carbohydrates they were feeding her to make her gain weight were actually killing her. The tragic irony.

Using my newly honed triage skills, I began suggesting everyone get tested for celiac disease. I made phone calls to family and friends, people whose family and health histories I already knew. I also annoyed many of these people, for which I am not apologizing. I suggested all four of my best friends from high school get tested. On a visit to Buffalo, I stayed (freeloaded) with one of my Irish friends and tried unsuccessfully to get her to agree to a cheek swab for the genetic testing. She adamantly refused, but her lovely Italian husband jumped in and said he would like to do the test. Knowing his family medical history, I thought that was a grand idea, so cheek-swab him we did. In a few weeks, his test came back positive for HLA-DQ2. We talked about the ramifications of being a gene carrier. He stated he had a doctor's appointment because the doctor wanted to work him up for liver, kidney, and lung problems. Wow. I suggested he request that his doctor run a celiac blood panel along with all of the other labs.

Shortly after that, I received an email from him that basically stated, "My test is positive. I don't want celiac disease. What do I do now?"

I offered to fly back to Buffalo and get him squared away. I suggested it would be a great idea if he shared this information with his family and got his fabulous son tested, who suffered from eczema, projectile vomiting, colic, and a few other maladies as a baby. We had a long conversation. I explained the problematic recommendation of a duodenal biopsy and reminded him the only way he would have a positive blood test is if he had intestinal damage that very well could be missed on biopsy.

He called me back a few weeks later and told me he had gone ahead with the biopsy. "Good news," he said. "The doctor said I don't have celiac disease."

I stewed about this for a moment while holding on the line. My response came out of my mouth in true Tourette's form: "I guess you found a doctor that told you what you wanted to hear."

These are the people I love and want to be healthy and live longer than I do. I selfishly want them to not be sick or develop cancer, autoimmune issues, or any number of other debilitating diseases. Alcoholics and drug abusers and gluten addle-brained people are all in the same category. The crossover is compelling. More and more commonly, people are coming into to my office or calling for a consultation because they are ready to feel better or because they finally got diagnosed with celiac disease. Occasionally, both men and women have come in and said, "Just tell me what to do and how to eat and I will listen to you, because nothing else has helped and I am tired of feeling/being sick." These people are motivated.

One of the important lessons I am still learning, though, is that I can't fix people if they don't want to be fixed. In the past, when confronted with patients who were reluctant to take my advice, my New York/emergency department/redhead bitchy nurse self would say things like, "That's fine, obviously you like being sick." Or, "Don't call me when you have bowel cancer. I am telling you that just because you have a strong family history of bowel cancer, you don't have to expect to get it too. It is preventable."

Now trust me: I have not been silenced, and my enthusiasm has not been tempered at all, but I am also learning to be quiet and listen. One of my dear friends and mentors, a fabulous naturopathic doctor and former school teacher, Lisa Shaver, once advised me to perhaps instead ask people, "How is what you are doing working for you? Is it perhaps time to try something different?"

Like I said, I'm learning.

Dangerous? No, *You're* Dangerous!

In the fall of 2007, I made the decision to take advantage of my health insurance that would pay for me to be seen anywhere. Apparently, though, there were no doctors in Oregon or on the West Coast who specialized in celiac disease, so I decided to go to the Columbia University Celiac Disease Center, where Dr. Peter Green is the director.

I made my appointment, got preapproved by the insurance company, and was informed by the office staff that even though I had insurance and had been preapproved, I would have to pay $500 cash the day of my appointment and then be reimbursed by my insurance company. What? I made several dozen phone calls, because this made no sense to me whatsoever. I had insurance coverage, I had been preapproved, and I wanted that to work the way it is supposed to work: without my having to fork over $500 to see the doctor and wait to get my money back. Then I found out my appointment would not be with Dr. Green but with another GI doc specializing in celiac disease. Fine.

So, the morning of my appointment, I was ready. I had pulled as much cash as I could out of the ATM the day before. I leapt on the subway that I was sure would exit me at the doorsteps of the hospital that housed the Columbia University Celiac Disease Center. I thought I knew which subway train to take to get there. Nope. I exited from below ground, then looked up expecting to see a big hospital-like structure, but nothing resembling a hospital was in clear view. I had no idea where I was, which, as you'll know if this has ever happened to you, is very disorienting. I had that "where the hell am I" look on my face and was spinning around looking at street signs or any signs that would give me a sense of where I was and how to get where I wanted to go.

With a complete trust in the kindness of strangers, I stopped the first person I could reliably focus on as I came out of my "I am lost" stupor. He was the kindest man. He took me to the bus stop, waited with me, told the bus driver where I wanted to go, and confirmed where I needed to get a transfer. The bus driver had me sit in the front, and repeated which transfers to take and where to exit the bus. I felt completely stupid for getting lost but also extremely thankful to these sweet New York men for getting me to my destination. I am always thankful for my habit of leaving early for an appointment, in case of delay or getting on the wrong bus or train.

When I exited the bus, lo and behold, there was the hospital I had been expecting to see when I had first exited the subway. I found Harkness Pavilion, located the ATM, withdrew another couple hundred dollars and took the elevator up to the designated floor.

I was somewhat shocked and surprised to see the conditions in which the celiac disease center was operating. To say "cramped and antiquated" would be the least of it. There were four or five receptionists, and their desks were crammed into the smallest office I had ever seen. I handed over my money to the woman I now felt I had a special relationship with because we had already spoken on the phone so many times about my insurance issues. I once again voiced my concerns that I had insurance, before I handed over the wad of bills, and she kindly asked me what insurance was it that I had? I told her the name of the insurance company and she said she had never heard of it, so they wouldn't bill the insurance and I had to pay cash. I then felt compelled to tell her that even though I lived three thousand miles away, I still lived in the contiguous United States. This made no sense to me then, nor does it make any sense to me now.

I checked in, sat down on a bench in the hallway, and waited my turn to be called. After being called, I was taken to a small exam room. The doctor entered, sat down and started interviewing me. I explained how I came to be here and that I didn't have a formal diagnosis of celiac disease and why. I then explained that I was a nurse and was telling people to consider a gluten-free diet, whether they could get tested or not.

She looked at me like I had lost my mind, and rather grumpily told me that what I was doing was "dangerous." Huh? I further explained that there was no celiac disease center where I lived, or anywhere on the West Coast, for that matter, and we were also lacking in any doctors who would order celiac panels. Plus, the false negative rate of the antibody testing was notoriously high, some had estimated 70 percent, a fact I certainly understood with my own falsely negative tests.

"What if these people really had celiac disease and decided not to stay on a gluten-free diet?" she asked. "And if these people opted not to stay on a gluten-free diet because they didn't know they had celiac disease," she said, I was potentially causing harm. "What if the people that were not getting proper testing were really celiac and they didn't know that? What if they started a gluten-free diet but didn't stay on it because they didn't have an official diagnosis?"

I did not see it that way, and I still to this day do not subscribe to that point of view, not in the least. Plenty of people have a biopsy-confirmed diagnosis of celiac disease, and they still choose to be haphazard with their diet. In my opinion, withholding important information and making testing difficult or even impossible to obtain is much more dangerous. I do, however, always recommend people get tested before they go on a gluten-free diet, just in case it is positive and so they at least have some sort of baseline test. So we had a bit of a spirited conversation during my appointment about the "dangers" of suggesting a gluten-free diet to people without "proper" testing.

After our discussion was over, I put on my little gown, fully exposing my still-bloomed DH and my recovering body, and sat on the exam table waiting for her to return. I was thinking the whole time, I should have taken all of that cash and seen a few Broadway plays instead of coming here. Oh, well. I'm here now, so I might as well see this adventure through to the end.

Then she quizzed me on my rash. "Did I have blisters?"

Sometimes, but they were quickly scratched away.

"Was it painful?"

Yes.

"Was it itchy?"

Horribly.

"Humph."

She drew and spun my blood herself (not even a lab tech!) right there in the room. For this, she gets a passing grade for her phlebotomy skills. She then ordered up a long list of lab tests, including a celiac panel. I had at this point been on a gluten-free diet for a year and expected it to be negative, especially considering my first antibody test had been negative. Hmmm.

We finished up that less than pleasant or productive appointment, after which I was offered the opportunity to see the registered dietitian at the Columbia Celiac Disease Center. This offer I thought long and hard about. I had already seen dietitians and nutritionists—number one, whom my insurance did not cover, even though celiac disease is a diet change only. And number two—no offense to nutritionists or RDs in general—who were the opposite of helpful during any of my appointments with them. One dietitian showed me plastic fruit, told me to eat low-fat foods, and suggested I order a tome listing all of the gluten-free food products on the market, which would be updated with new pages every few months or so. Again, not helpful. But since I was already in the esteemed halls of the Columbia University Celiac Disease Center and it was only going to cost me another $150 to see the registered dietitian, I agreed to do so, halfheartedly. It was the best decision I've ever made.

I met with Anne Roland-Lee, RD, who was not what I anticipated or expected at all. First of all, in keeping with the interesting setup, we had our appointment in what appeared also to be the staff's break room. At one point, Dr. Green himself appeared, excused the interruption, asked Anne a question, then left again.

At that moment, I was a bit star struck—the author of THE book on celiac disease!—but I would get over that rather quickly. Anne, I decided after my appointment with her, was the real rock star. She did not talk to me about food. Rather, her first question was, "Tell me about your family."

I was dumbfounded. "Why? What do you want to know? I am only genetically related to my son, since I birthed him."

"Test him," she said.

"My [now ex-] husband, a late-onset type 1 diabetic at the age of 32?"

"Test him."

"My daughter, Hannah, is African-American; she is adopted."

"Test her," she said.

"There is a girl who came to live with us when she was eighteen years old. She's short, red haired, neurotic as hell, and lives in New York City."

"Oh my God, test her too," she said.

My paternal grandfather, Felix, died in February 1969 when I was three years old. He worked in a bakery, had "baker's asthma," and died at the age of sixty of kidney failure. My maternal grandfather, Milford, died in April 1970, also at the age of sixty, when I was four years old, of alcoholism and pernicious anemia, a B12 deficiency. All of my great aunts and uncles on my mother's side also had bowed legs. As a child, I thought that was caused by riding horses too long before there were cars. Now that I know they all had rickets, I see rickets every day and everywhere. If you look for it, you will too. Rickets is caused by a deficiency in vitamin D, a fat-soluble vitamin. In toddlerhood, when a child is learning to walk, if the child is deficient in vitamin D, along with magnesium and calcium, then the bones in the legs are soft and unable to support the weight of the torso and head, so the legs bow. I am a very firm believer that rickets should be illegal, especially in the United States, but it isn't.

A genogram is a tool to look at the medical health of your family to identify trends and assess risk for addictions, cancer and other diseases. A genogram using my family on both sides screamed celiac disease when viewed through that lens. At this point, I just assumed my whole family had undiagnosed celiac disease, especially the ones with personality disorders, addiction issues and early death. So I made contact with Kimball Genetics in Denver, Colorado, and started getting my family tested for the celiac genes. My son is HLA-DQ2.5 positive. My now ex-husband Brad, a late-onset insulin-dependent diabetic at the age of thirty-two, is HLA-DQ8 positive. My African-American daughter is HLA-DQ2 positive. The short, red-haired, neurotic-as-hell who lives in NYC is HLA-DQ2 homozygous. I am HLA-DQ2.5 homozygous. The genetic testing revealed that we were ALL predisposed genetically and at risk for developing celiac disease. Wow. How does that happen? How could that be? I wondered: are there just so many of us who are gene carriers that we can't help but find each other, or are we drawn to each other on a very basic genetic level? Fascinating.

I am all about common sense, which it turns out, is not so common. If you consume a food or a beverage and it makes you sick or causes you harm, don't eat or drink it. Sometimes we, or our bodies, or more commonly as we are discovering, our microbiome, craves foods or substances that are bad for us. We need to consciously make that distinction through elimination diets, challenges (never, ever intentionally with gluten), and sometimes specific testing. I also have no power over what people choose to eat. None. I can give people the information, teach them why they are reacting, and point out the genetics involved, but at the end of the day, I cannot nor would I ever follow people around and say, "Don't eat that; it's not gluten free." That would be weird, and my life would suck. You determine what you eat, and sometimes that is a hard job. Sometimes, it's the most important job of your life. So take this job seriously, and choose your food wisely. But if you ask me about your food choices, I will tell you the truth, so don't get pissed at me. You asked me.

My gluten-free diet is very different from what most people would consider a gluten-free diet. In the beginning, when I was starting out, I made choices that I assumed were reasonable on a gluten-free diet. My learning curve was incredibly steep. But it wasn't long before I was thinking critically about the food-as-medicine I was relying on to heal my very damaged body. Saying it's "gluten free" is not a comforting statement to make to me anymore. I rely on my knowledge base to decide if what is put in front of me is truly gluten free or if I am going to risk a possible exposure by eating it. Plus, there is the added threat of cross-contamination from well-intentioned food preparers, whether professional restaurant staff, family and friends, or the community at large, who don't know beans about what gluten is, where it hides, and how even a breadcrumb or a dusting of flour will poison me for months. Our local sushi restaurant, which I love because they only use fresh crab, not "krab" (made with wheat), insists on putting their gluten-free tamari in a container labeled and made for regular, wheat-containing soy sauce, and just writing a big "GF" on the lid in permanent marker. Nope. I am not touching that with a ten-foot pole. I either bring my own bottle or some packets, or (as I am learning to do) just enjoy my sushi and sashimi sans sauce.

And food itself is not the only danger we need to have on our radar. I am always leery of people in a perceived position of authority or power who attempt to exert scientific evidence as a weapon of mass destruction over a population that is not bending to the will of the propagators of misinformation: *Don't worry your pretty little head about the science because you are too dumb to understand what I, the doctor, am telling you to do.* Are you old enough to remember snake oil salesmen? Always ask yourself, "Is this doctor trying to sell me a product?" Does the doctors' research support the development of a product? A pill? Does it smell fishy but it isn't a fish oil capsule? (And if that fish oil is fresh, it shouldn't smell fishy either.) Does the doctor disclose any financial ties to pharmaceutical corporations? Do you know what that means? Magic cures? Tonics? Prescription medications? Pharmaceuticals are enormous corporations that make enormous amounts of money from selling drugs. Period. To whom do they sell those drugs? Sick people. They love sick people who can't or don't ask questions and who just "trust" that the doctor has their best interests at heart.

Doctors get paid whether they do a good job or not. What is the incentive to do a good job? You might say, "Well, if they don't do a good job, then the doctors get sued." Really? By whom? Dead people don't sue. And already traumatized, grieving and victimized family and friends usually don't sue either. Suing the doctor isn't going to undo the damage or bring loved ones back to life, but it could take away the doctor's chance to maim or kill that next person. I hear a multitude of excuses from patients, some of whom are nurses and doctors themselves, as to why they won't sue a doctor for negligence. But even if they're unsure or afraid of what to do about it, the bottom line is that people are tired of being lied to, misled, and mistreated, sometimes for years.

The Excuses

There is no point in talking to people who are angry or skeptical until they themselves get thoroughly tested for celiac disease and they know their current status. That said, I most assuredly love to discuss gluten intolerance and celiac disease, even with the most ardent skeptic and/or scientifically minded individual. My only request to these skeptical, scientifically minded people is that if they really want to have a conversation or a debate about gluten intolerance and celiac disease, that they please do some research beforehand.

If they are adults and refuse to get tested, fine. But if they have children, they must get those children tested. These children should not have to suffer for the ignorance of their parents. One of the issues I hear repeatedly is that one parent feeds the children gluten free or according to their specific dietary requirements, but the other parent, sometimes an ex-spouse, will ignore the dietary restrictions and feed the child whatever they want to feed them, sometimes intentionally making the child sick. If this is not already a legal issue, it very quickly will be, as this behavior is abusive and neglectful. Would these parents withhold insulin from a diabetic child in order to get back at their ex-spouse? Then I have to remind them that at this time in history with our current testing options, you can be ruled in but you can't be ruled out, ever.

If you keep in mind that gluten is addictive, it is easy to see why people behave so vehemently and protectively of their right to eat it. They sound like Gollum from *The Lord of the Rings: "MY PRECIOUS..."* Having previously been one of those unpleasant people who would have said any and all of the statements listed below, I completely understand the addiction, devotion, and unwillingness to give up gluten or dairy or any other foods that are causing harm. I understand completely.

But, without further ado:

The Excuses

• *You people are crazy. You honestly think nobody should eat gluten?! You will have to pry my bread, my pasta and yes, my GLUTEN out of my cold dead hands. I would never go on a gluten-free diet—I LOVE gluten.* • *I eat gluten free during the week but on the weekends, I love my beer* • *I'm a gluten-aholic. I'm a carb-aholic. I'm addicted to wheat.* • *I went on a gluten-free diet once and I got so sick I had to quit.* (Detoxing, perhaps?) *I felt worse on a gluten-free diet.* • *My body needs grains. That's why they call it comfort food, right? I eat macaroni and cheese, pizza, grilled cheese sandwiches, spaghetti noodles with butter.* • *Wheat and dairy. Wheat and dairy. Wheat and dairy and more wheat and dairy.* • *But isn't it all good for me?* • *I've been eating gluten my entire life. I'm not changing now.* • *I don't have that problem with gluten.* • *I don't have celiac disease. I was tested once and I don't have it.* • *I can eat whatever I want. I have an iron stomach.* (This was ME!) • *My sister/mother/brother/uncle/grandmother/cousin etc. has celiac disease but I don't have the same symptoms they have, so, therefore I don't have it and the doctor said I don't need to get tested.* • *My doctor won't test me because he doesn't believe in it.* • *My doctor thinks it's a fad.* • *My doctor won't test me because I don't have diarrhea.* • *I'm overweight. My doctor says fat people can't be celiac.* • *My daughter/son is growing fine and smart so I know he/she can't have it. Look at her. She's so healthy. She doesn't need to be on a special diet.* • *I got diagnosed with a "wheat allergy"/celiac when I was a baby, but my parents were told I grew out of it.* • *I was sick all of the time and took a ton of antibiotics when I was young for throat and ear infections. I had no immune system when I was a kid, but I'm better now.*

Celiac: The Sneaky Shapeshifter

Once my rash disappeared on my hands, it started showing up on the rest of my body in funky, itchy, painful patches. It goes without saying that if you have a rash on your skin, it's visible for all to see. It can become hard to cover the rash as it spreads. Everything irritates the rash. It's embarrassing. Shaving, pedicures, manicures, dresses, skirts, bikinis, shorts, all become things from the past, from before the rash exploded.

So I began to read every dermatology book, journal article, and website I could for possible clues. On my breaks from work in the emergency departments, I would go to the hospital libraries and dive into the archives of books on dermatology. The answer had to be hidden somewhere in all of those resources, and I was determined to find it.

But I wasn't able to self-diagnose, because dermatitis herpetiformis is misrepresented in every dermatology book I have ever read. Dermatitis herpetiformis was named as such because the lesions were noted as resembling a viral herpes lesion. But DH is not a viral lesion, nor is it related to herpes; it just looks similar to those lesions. DH occurs when IgA deposits appear underneath the skin in order to work themselves out of the body, as does any other toxin you ingest. DH has also been directly connected to celiac disease since 1967. It has been confirmed by many practitioners worldwide that if you have DH, you have celiac disease. While DH manifests on the surface of your body, the deep tissues are also involved. DH is merely an external expression of what is happening internally. If you have a chronic rash, especially one such as DH, you have damage to other organs —primarily intestinal damage in the form of villous atrophy, but most likely other organ damage as well.

Think meth "bugs"—you know, all of those sores that meth abusers get on their skin because they use methamphetamine, a poison, and then they see crystals or bugs or worms crawling out of their skin, causing them to pick at their skin. The nice thing for meth users is that it doesn't take very long for the meth toxins to clear once they stop using meth. They may always have pitted, scarred skin, their teeth have rotted, and they have no friends or money, but the rash clears up. If you have DH, the good news is the only treatment necessary is a diet change. The bad news is it can take up to ten years for the IgA deposits to work themselves out of your body by way of your integumentary system, your skin. For those of us who suffer with DH, it is very disconcerting that gluten is a much stronger toxin than meth (which I have never, ever used).

Many articles and even "expert" resources will tell you it doesn't matter what you put on your skin, that the gluten proteins are too large to get through your skin and to your intestines to cause damage. If you're reacting to something, it's not the gluten, but rather something else in that product, some other irritant. This is what I hear and have read from reputable sources. I will tell you, though, that it *absolutely* matters what you put on your skin. Your skin is your largest organ, and it takes roughly twenty-six seconds for whatever you put on your skin to enter your bloodstream. If you're applying mascara with wheat germ oil as an ingredient—who puts wheat germ oil in mascara?! Many cosmetic manufacturers do, because it is the cheapest oil—you are putting that wheat germ oil in direct contact with your mucous membranes; therefore, it takes even *less* than twenty-six seconds to enter the bloodstream.

If you are gluten intolerant or celiac, you may be sensitive to *anything* to do with wheat, barley, rye, and oats. It is not just the "gluten" component—the gliadin, hordein, secalin, and avenin proteins themselves—that can cause harm; it is potentially any component of these grains. Not only are wheat germ oil, hydrolyzed wheat germ proteins, or hydrolyzed barley protein usually contaminated with gluten, but many of us are sensitized to every component of these grains.

One patient was buying a lotion product faithfully because it didn't cause her to break out in a rash when she used it. When she ran out of that tube, she went to the store and bought a replacement tube. But shortly after using the new tube, her skin started breaking out again. She brought both the old and the new tubes of lotion to my office. After carefully reading and comparing the reading the ingredient lists, the only difference we found was that the new tube had hydrolyzed oat protein in it. The oat protein was causing the skin reaction. She stopped using the "new formula" and her rash cleared up.

I remember trying desperately to use over-the-counter products that were specifically marketed to people with itchy, sensitive skin. Many of them are grain based. No wonder none of them ever relieved any of my symptoms, and usually made my rashes worse. I was placing my hope, trust, and money in products that were merely adding poison in the form of wheat, barley, and oats directly onto my rashes, which were unknowingly caused by my daily consumption of wheat, barley, rye and oats. The mystery is solved.

When I was thirteen years old, I finally got chickenpox. The older you are when you get chickenpox, the worse it is, and mine was a textbook case of bad. I was covered from head to toe, in my mouth, ears, and, well, everywhere with blisters. What is the medically recommended treatment for chickenpox? Oatmeal baths! I missed several days of school, cried for days, and suffered through the agony with the help of over-the-counter medications for itching and sleep. My skin still sports the divots and scars from that intensely painful episode. I can assure you that if you've never had dermatitis herpetiformis, you don't ever want it. It's like having the worst case of chickenpox ever, all of the time. As noted by Lionel Fry, an emeritus professor of dermatology, one unnamed sufferer described dermatitis herpetiformis as such: "...like rolling in stinging nettles naked with a sunburn, then wrapping yourself in a wool blanket filled with ants and fleas..."

When I read that, I thought, yes, that is exactly the description of how bad my skin, my largest organ, felt day in and day out, for years. If no one was at home when I stepped into the shower, I would scream out loud when the water hit my skin. If my family was at home, I would produce the silent scream. I have read in multiple references to DH that it was not uncommon for people to commit suicide because there was no relief from the maddeningly intense itch and searing pain. I can't tell you how many times as both a child and an adult I have been admonished for scratching my skin, because "that'll just make it worse." Not really. I'm not sure how it could have been worse.

Despite all of the scratching, one of the remarkable characteristics of my DH is that it rarely bleeds. As a matter of fact, there were a few times, when my body was really starting to shut down, that I noticed even when I cut myself by accident, I didn't bleed. Apparently, this was happening because my body was shunting all of my blood to my core organs and my brain. No perfusion to my periphery—my arms, legs, fingers, or toes—so I didn't bleed. At least I saved money on Band-Aids.

Initially, upon my diagnosis with DH and celiac disease, Dr. Haberman, my dermatologist, offered a prescription for Dapsone, an early antibiotic, which somehow suppresses the DH, but also can cause hemolytic anemia, neuropathy, liver damage, bone damage, cancer, and a few other unpleasant side effects, so it is recommended to take it only for a short period of time. After quickly researching Dapsone, I opted not to take it at all and to treat my DH with only a gluten-free diet. Of course, you would also have to go immediately on a gluten-free diet anyway even if you decided to take the Dapsone. I have heard stories from patients over the years, though, in which instead of being put on both Dapsone AND a gluten-free diet, many patients were only prescribed Dapsone and not advised to go gluten free. These people would report, "I have to take the Dapsone. I've been taking it for years—otherwise, that dang rash comes back!" Not shockingly, several of these people had developed liver failure, cancer, and some of those other noted bad side effects.

In addition to the relationship between celiac disease and skin conditions, an area of study that is absolutely exploding with new information is everything to do with the neurological components of celiac disease. The gut-brain connection relies in large part on the vagus nerve, which runs from our brains directly to our intestines. This nerve is a great transporter of information, primarily from our guts to our brains. We know when we are hungry because we feel hunger in our guts, which transmits neurotransmitters from our intestines to our brains telling us to eat. The flow of information, however, is not as good the other way around. Your brain is not as effective when attempting to communicate with your intestines.

An interesting phenomenon I have recently noticed occurring in my own still-healing body is that shortly after experiencing a low-grade headache, I will experience some unpleasant bowel disturbance. Thankfully, I do not nor did I ever suffer from migraines. But did you know there is a condition called abdominal migraines? I believe Western medicine is missing the boat on migraine headaches, what causes them, and how we treat them. The neurological signs and symptoms of celiac disease can present in many other forms too, including difficulty swallowing, gluten ataxia or difficulty walking straight, gastroparesis, seizure disorders, peripheral neuropathies, psychiatric disorders, anxiety, schizophrenia, and many more.

There is an astounding amount of research literature linking neuropsychiatric disorders with gluten intolerance and celiac disease. I have given eight-hour lectures on the neurological and mental health components related to undiagnosed gluten intolerance and celiac disease. Dr. Marios Hadjivassiliou, a clinical senior lecturer at the University of Sheffield in the UK and a consultant neurologist at Sheffield Teaching Hospitals NHS Foundation Trust and Chesterfield Royal Hospital, is someone who is running full steam ahead regarding the study and documentation of patients affected neurologically by celiac disease. He is my hero, and I enormously admire the work he is doing because 1) as far as I know, he doesn't take any pharmaceutical money which could potentially influence research outcomes, 2) he has appreciation for the fact that many more patients present with neurological complements of celiac disease than with gastrointestinal symptoms, and 3) many of these patients aren't meeting the current criteria of celiac disease but still test positive for gluten intolerance utilizing the AGA and anti-tissue transglutaminase 6 antibody testing (along with exhibiting symptoms, sometimes exclusively in the nervous system).

One of the most fascinating and compelling research articles on the celiac-neurological overlap to be published recently was one by Dr. Reidun Stenberg entitled "Anti-Transglutaminase 6

Antibodies in Children and Young Adults with Cerebral Palsy." Dr. Stenberg and her researchers compared the prevalence of anti-TG6 antibodies in child patients with cerebral palsy (CP) to a control group, and found that there was a significantly higher level of anti-TG6 antibodies in the children with CP. They found that the kids with CP "do not have a higher prevalence of celiac disease than expected in the regional population but they do have more frequent immunoreactivity to gluten and other dietary food components compared to matched controls." So children with CP may not have a higher incidence of celiac disease proper, but they are still reacting neurologically to the gliadin protein.

I had the honor and privilege of meeting and talking with Dr. Stenberg at two of the conferences hosted by the Columbia University Celiac Disease Center. Dr. Stenberg explained the results of this study to me during one of our conversations. I was enthralled by her brilliance in investigating gluten intolerance and celiac disease in the cerebral palsy population—but also confused. I point-blank asked her WHY she thought to study gluten intolerance and celiac disease in this particular population.

Her answer was stunningly altruistic. "We have a group of children and adults that can't speak for themselves. They rely on people to speak for them and to advocate for them."

Dr. Stenberg is truly one of my heroes. It makes me weepy to know there are doctors and researchers who are engaged in the scientific process for the benefit of our most vulnerable populations and not just for their own benefit. I give a standing ovation to Dr. Stenberg, Dr. Hadjivassiliou, Pascale Aeschlimann, Nigel Hoggard, Daniel Aeschlimann, and the rest of the research teams doing this kind of work.

It is also well established that gluten intolerance and celiac disease are capable of causing decreased oxygen flow in the body. As a child, about nine years old, I vividly remember watching my Uncle Jim play cards, usually rummy, with all of my other relatives, and looking at his hands—and in particular his fingernails. I found it interesting that my uncle, a lifelong chain smoker with a barrel chest, and one of the funniest and nicest guys I had ever met, had large, spoon-shaped fingernails—and I had them too.

This had been filed away in my brain for years until I went to nursing school and discovered there is a name for our wide fingernails: clubbing, which is an indicator of hypoperfusion or decreased blood supply and therefore, oxygen supply to the tissues. My uncle was a lifelong smoker. I, at the age of nine, was not a smoker. I did, however, already have the purple-pallor hands of someone with Raynaud's phenomenon. Again, I thought this was because I lived in Buffalo where most of the time it was very cold. I had no idea at the time that Raynaud's is an autoimmune issue that causes hypoperfusion or a decreased oxygen supply to the fingers, toes, and other tissues, leading to clubbed fingernails. Because of the eczema, the Raynaud's, and my use of steroid creams, my chances of ever being a hand model were nipped in the bud.

Where else is perfusion of tissues a concern in celiac disease? Well, come to find out through the work of Dr. Hadjivassiliou, it turns out that our brains get hypoperfused too. There are several things our brain needs to function appropriately, and one of those things happens to be oxygen. Your brain requires and utilizes at least 25 percent of all of the oxygen in the blood. If your brain doesn't have access to enough oxygen, such as when you are climbing a mountain, you may experience sleepiness, apathy, and impaired judgment. Brain fog explained.

Now let's make a leap—and for men, this isn't much of a leap at all. If your brain is hypoperfused, and potentially other organs in your body as well, my theory is that erectile dysfunction is caused by decreased blood flow and hypoperfusion to the penis. Now, if the hypoperfusion is potentially related to eating gluten—leading to a hypoxic state in the brain, as has been shown by Dr. Hadjivassiliou and other researchers—then treating erectile dysfunction with a gluten-free diet certainly makes sense to me.

So let's add all men with erectile dysfunction to the list of people to be tested for gluten intolerance and celiac disease, shall we? This may not be good news for the makers of Cialis and Viagra, thanks to the nearly fifteen million prescriptions written for these drugs between October 2013 and September 2014. But think of all of the happy couples that discover after reading this book that once they both go gluten free (remember that a significant cause of cross-contamination is through bodily fluids, which includes semen), the man has ALL of his facilities up and operational, so to speak, including his brain. This may very possibly be a boon to women as well due to the similar nature of the process. I am not a sex scientist, but I believe this is a study just begging to be researched.

When Gluten Free Is Not Enough (Love Your Farmers and Pay Them Too)

After I had been on a gluten-free, dairy-free, soy-free diet for four years and was not only still alive but significantly healthier, I decided to celebrate by participating in another marathon. Prior to that, I had completed the Dublin marathon in 1998 with several of my emergency nurse cohorts. I had agreed that I would run a marathon, which I had never dreamed I could do, IF I could go to Ireland. So we all trained, flew to Ireland, visited the Guinness Museum, drank more than our fair share of Guinness well before I knew I was celiac, toured the countryside, and ran in the marathon.

I have no illusions about being a fast runner. In my thoughts and dreams, I am speedy and run like the wind. In reality, not so much speed at all; much more plodding and a fair amount of putting one foot in front of the other. I am not a winner; I am a finisher. It may take me several hours, but I will finish—again, those tenacious Polish genes that drive me and keep me going, until the finish line or the end. By the spring of 2011, I had already finished two Portland Marathons, been on two super-fun Hood to Coast Relay teams, and finished several half marathons and many shorter races. I may not have been fast, but I take a fair amount of pride out of the fact that I participated and always finished.

In May of that year, I had started seeing a new doctor in town and decided to make her my primary care provider. It is my practice to not refer people to new practitioners until I check them out first myself. So I made an appointment and went to see her. The doctor, Keri Erland, MD, was very thorough. She ordered the tests I was requesting and added a few more, one being an antinuclear antibody titer (ANA) panel, which tests for autoimmune issues. I wasn't at all worried about being positive because I figured all of my autoimmune issues had been resolved on my gluten-, dairy-, and soy-free diet.

My vitamin D level was low despite taking supplements, and my B12 level of 396 was on the low end of the normal range. But when my ANA came back positive with a titer of 1:160 (with < 1:40 being negative), and an ANA pattern referenced as "speckled," which is associated with systemic lupus erythema (SLE), Sjögren's syndrome, scleroderma, polymyositis, rheumatoid arthritis, and other connective tissue autoimmune diseases, I was really unhappy. I knew I had been symptomatic for at least seven autoimmune diseases before I went gluten free, but because many of the symptoms had disappeared, I thought the diseases themselves had resolved. I was not amused. How could it possibly be positive? And why were my vitamin D3 and B12 levels still so low?

Dr. Erland advised me to make an appointment with a rheumatologist, and to call soon, because it takes so long to get an appointment with a rheumatologist.

"Why does it take so long?" I asked.

"Because there are so many people with autoimmune diseases that the rheumatologists are very busy," she said.

Did anyone think to ask, I pondered, why so many people have autoimmune diseases? Dr. Erland also informed me that I was going to have to take medications like Remicade and Imuran for the rest of my life. I firmly and resoundingly informed her that I was not going to take those medications. She told me that I needed to make an appointment with the rheumatologist and then decide what to do.

I remember going home with the test results, shuffling the papers, researching the results, contemplating the ramifications of a positive test, and being seriously depressed. Then one night while I was sleeping and blissfully unconscious, I was rudely awakened by intense pain in the right proximal joint of my second digit, my pointer finger. At first, I thought that someone had broken into my house and somehow managed to break my finger while I was sleeping. As I slowly regained a semblance of consciousness, I still thought someone had broken my finger, it hurt that bad, but nothing made sense.

I sat up in bed, grumpily turned on the light, and realized my finger wasn't broken, but that the joint sure was swollen and painful to flex or extend. How could my finger hurt like it was broken but not actually BE broken? Regardless, having my pointer finger in that much pain with limited movement was pretty much a debilitating injury for a knitter. Heck, it would have made it hard to drive, dress myself, or even type.

So, later that morning, I took myself to immediate care and saw my friend and colleague, Dr. Chee Lee, whom I adored until he took another job in Florida and moved away. I explained my situation with my painful finger joint. Dr. Lee sent me for an x-ray of both hands, presuming there would be radiographic indicators of arthritis in that joint. He also opted to order lab work, which included another ANA. I explained to him that I'd had a positive ANA test in May, and had come back with a "speckled pattern." This time, the results again came back positive, and this confirmatory second test did not make me happy, not at all. Dr. Lee advised me to make an appointment with my primary care doctor for follow-up and gave me a sample of an arthritis anti-inflammatory medication, which I took exactly one of. The pain resolved and thankfully did not return, ever.

But the whole episode got me thinking and rethinking some things, so it was at this point that I decided to change my diet again to a Paleo diet. My friends Cain and Tammy Credicott had already made the transition from gluten, dairy, soy, egg and nut free to a Paleo lifestyle, which in addition to no gluten or dairy removes ALL grains, including rice and corn, as well as legumes, which includes peanuts and beans. Cain had recently started a new business venture called *Paleo Magazine*, and Tammy had already authored my favorite gluten-free cookbook, *The Healthy Gluten Free Life*, and was now working on Paleo cookbooks. They had encouraged me before to think about leaping into a Paleo diet, but I gave them the same mamby-pamby lame excuses and whiny "I have already had to give up so much" and "I can't do that too" and whatever other cheesy justifications I hear frequently. "I am too busy, blah blah blah. I can't possibly do that!"

At this point, though, I was highly motivated due to the second positive ANA panel, and I leapt onto the Paleo train full steam ahead. At first, I once again struggled to figure out what to eat.

But very quickly, I learned the basics of sticking to grass-fed, no-antibiotics, no-hormones beef and lamb, free-range poultry, wild fish, organic fruits and vegetables, and tree nuts and seeds. I read labels, and quickly adopted a couple of basic rules for buying anything in a package. One, the product must be manufactured in a designated gluten-free facility. Two, there must be no more than five ingredients in the product. I will fudge on this rule occasionally, especially when there is a Hail Merry Meyer Lemon tart involved. I must also be able to picture what those ingredients are; I know what a cashew, a cranberry, a date, and a pumpkin seed look like. I have no idea what hydrolyzed vegetable protein looks like nor do I know what it is made from. What is natural flavoring? Where does it come from? The second I can't answer those basic questions, that product goes immediately back up on the shelf and I don't buy it. I have no time to call 1-800 numbers only to get someone on the line who has no idea how to even spell gluten, let alone where the ingredients come from.

We as gluten-free consumers can be collectively very powerful—and I am voting with my dollars. Food companies need to be very transparent about the ingredients in their products, or I don't buy them. If I do buy a product, it is one researched and developed by a family or a person I can talk to if I need to. This amounts to accountability for the quality of the product. Once a small company has been bought out, it becomes very difficult to determine whether the manufacturing standards for their products have changed. Are their products still manufactured in a designated gluten-free facility, for instance? So once these small companies get bought by large corporations, and you know the ones, then I stop buying those products. These corporations get not one penny more of my hard-earned money, if I can help it.

As part of this new shift, I also finally came to understand the importance of a good high-fat diet, especially since I was celiac. The worst thing you could ever tell a celiac patient with intestinal damage is to go on a gluten-free, low-fat diet. No wonder so many celiac patients die within the first year of diagnosis! The children in the 1920s, '30s, '40s, and '50s were being diagnosed with celiac disease with a fecal fat test. These kids had steatorrhea or fatty stools; they couldn't absorb the fat in their diet because of villous atrophy, and therefore, they couldn't absorb any fat-soluble vitamins (A, D, E, or K), which meant they were thereby starving, literally to death. During those initial few months on a Paleo diet, my breakfasts consisted of four to six local organic eggs, a pound of bacon, and two to three avocados. I also went back to my grandmother's habit of keeping a bowl (well, she used a coffee can) of bacon fat or lard near the stove, and I used it for everything. Wahoo!

It was during this new phase of high-fat eating that I also developed a new hobby. Whenever hospitals would sponsor one of those health-screening fairs, I would go in and ask to have my lipid panel checked.

The first question was always, "Are you fasting?" to which I would respond, "No."

Then the nurses would ask me what I ate for breakfast, and I would tell them: "Four to six eggs, a pound of bacon, and two to three avocados."

They would look at me stunned and say, "We can't test your lipid panel—it'll be through the roof!"

I would assure them it was okay, go ahead and test it. Every time I get tested, my lipid panel comes back completely within normal limits. Every time. I learned early on that eating good fats are the key and essential to healing my damaged intestines and neurological symptoms. In addition to the good fats in my grass-fed, antibiotic- and hormone-free beef and lamb, I also buy most of my pork from a local farmer who feeds the pigs chestnuts, forage and kitchen scraps. When I buy bacon at the store, it is Niman Ranch or Beeler's. I save all of my bacon fat and use it to sauté vegetables and green leafies. If my bacon doesn't have enough bacon fat on it, I throw in more bacon fat. Avocados, olive oil, high-quality fish oils, and nut butters other than peanut butter, especially pumpkin seed butter, are all excellent sources of high-quality dietary fat. This is one very crucial fact I wish someone had told me immediately. Instead, the powers that be extol the gluten-free, low-fat diet "because once our intestines heal and we start eating all of those gluten-free products we are going to get fat." No wonder people are still sick on a gluten-free diet.

Also, my body needs meat protein. If I have to eat vegetarian on a trip, the first thing I eat on returning home is a pound (which is now twelve ounces) of bacon. No kidding. My body must have meat, and this is not an option. Don't get me wrong. My diet is loaded with fresh organic fruits and vegetables, but meat is mandatory. Frequently, I counsel people that if they want to get better, if they want their symptoms to improve, they have to go back to eating meat. Some of the unhealthiest people I work with are vegan or vegetarian. After they start to eat meat again, they get better, healthier. Our bodies have the enzymes to break down the proteins in meat. They do not have the enzymes to break down the proteins in wheat or grains, as has been established repeatedly.

After being on a Paleo diet for a year, I made an appointment with my PCP. (I had never made an appointment with the rheumatologist. Bad patient.) She ordered labs to be drawn before my appointment, which included another ANA panel, along with tests for hemoglobin A1c, erythrocyte sedimentation rate (ESR, a test used to evaluate inflammation), magnesium, B12, and vitamin D.

My ANA panel came back completely negative—not just lower, but completely negative. "This never happens," my doctor said. "Once you have a positive ANA panel, it never comes back negative. What have you been doing?"

All I did was change my diet, I told her. I stepped it up to a good, high-fat Paleo diet and that was it. Not only that, but my vitamin D was now a much healthier 60.

"Excellent," she wrote on my report.

Before educating myself about Paleo, I had no idea that I had to take my A, D, E, and K vitamins with fat in order for them to be absorbed into my body. Even though I was taking supplements, my levels were always low. My ESR number was now zero. Zero as in no inflammation. My B12 was now up to the other end of the range at 674, my magnesium was 2.1, and my HgA1c was 5.5.

As a closing note she wrote, "Looks great!"

Another outcome of this new approach was that I needed to go shopping for new pants. Shopping is not my favorite pastime, so I power-shop. Plus, as a former Catholic all-girls' school alumni who wore polyester pleated plaid skirts as part of our school's dress code, I like to stick with my "uniform" clothes. That way, I can just zoom into a store, pick out the same pants in every color available, try them on, make my purchases, and leave. This particular day was no different in my routine. I went in, picked out a pile of pants in size 8, went to the changing room, and put them on. They didn't fit. They were too big. I grabbed up the extra material and schlepped out of my dressing room.

I asked the woman who worked there, "What happened? Did they cut these wrong? I am a size 8 and these are way too big on me."

She said, "No, they didn't cut them wrong. Those are just too big for you[, silly]." She went back out and picked out several more pairs of pants that were between size 4 and 6. Amazing. I really hadn't lost a pound, since I still weighed roughly 140 pounds on my five-foot, nine-and-three-quarter-inch frame, but my body composition had changed dramatically. Bonus!

It was at this point that I also started to add Paleo topics to my expanding repertoire of lectures and classes. Any lecture I give on the Paleo lifestyle is very well attended, and the Paleo presentations are very much the most requested lecture topic that I enthusiastically now give all over the country, in small towns and at large conferences. The Paleo community is my community. These are my people. My favorite attribute of this community is the constant questioning of all of the information available, the practice of assessing, modifying, and reassessing again. Thinking critically and realizing that we do not fit into a "one size fits all" food paradigm are the traits I most agree with in the Paleo community. Remarkably this is also what nurses do, day in and day out.

Everyone is an individual. My variations of the Paleo diet are always under review and subject to change. I very much continue to recognize and utilize my food as my medicine. I am always learning, modifying, and considering variations in how, what, and why I eat. Choosing food is not a static process but a dynamic one that involves making informed decisions based on options, information, and resources. Make no mistake, I am a foodie. I love great food. And finally, my food is loving me back in ways I am only beginning to understand.

I live in the Willamette (Will-AM-ette) Valley in Oregon. Thankfully, this region is what I refer to as "Food Utopia." I live an hour away from the Pacific Ocean, so fresh fish and seafood are plentiful. We also have access to fresh, organic fruits and vegetables nearly year-round from farmers markets and our local co-ops. Many of our local farmers raise grass-fed, no-antibiotics and no-hormones beef, lamb, and poultry, and we happily thank and pay them for their efforts. Farmer Dave, the owner of La Mancha Farm, calls me at butcher time, confirms my order, and then after it is all packaged, delivers a quarter or a half of beef to my house. He then helps me load it all into my freezer. He also raises Berkshire pork, free range, which is amazing.

Sam's dad, a local farmer, also sells some of us grass-fed, no-antibiotic, no-hormones beef for two dollars a pound. That's crazy, right? When we ask him why he sells it to us so cheaply, he responds, "Listen, I buy a few calves, put them out in the pasture. They mow the pasture for me, it costs me nothing to feed them. Plus, I sell the beef to people I love and I want them to eat healthy and well."

Happy, healthy cows and happy, healthy people. That said—and I am forever thankful for Sam's dad—I will happily pay more money to my local farmers for organic local food. I am much closer to my food now, and I know exactly where it comes from. I recognize its importance in my life. As a result, I want my farmers to make more than a living wage. I want them to be happy and healthy too. Nothing makes me unhappier than to hear someone at the farmers' market trying to get eggs or some produce for less than it is marked. Pay the farmers more than they are asking for their eggs. Give them a tip for getting up early, loading up their vehicles with produce and a stand, and standing out in the cold for hours. Pay them extra. Cheap food is not the bargain we thought it was.

Cheap "filler" food has been killing us slowly. Pay the farmers more and reap the health benefits of being stronger, healthier, and smarter, plus your money stays in the local economy. Bonus all around. My local farmers are my new best friends.

Portland, Oregon, which is an hour and a half north of where I live, is a gluten-free/Paleo mecca for safe, fabulous food. There are several excellent designated gluten-free bakeries there that I love to visit. New Cascadia Traditions Gluten Free Bakery offers their fabulous gluten free breads, bagels (!), and granola. Tula's Bakery has to-die-for chocolate chip cookies with sea salt, and savory pies. Kyra's Bake Shop in Lake Oswego is owned by Kyra, the three-time winner of *Cupcake Wars* on the Food Network for her world-famous gluten-free cupcakes. Petunia's Pies and Pastries has multitudes of 100 percent gluten-free/vegan sweet treats. When visiting Portland, it's not uncommon for me to have dessert first, on occasion, thanks to this abundance (and the fact I no longer have a yeast overgrowth).

Elsewhere in Portland, the Cultured Caveman started out as three food carts but recently opened up a brick-and-mortar restaurant that serves the most amazing Paleo food, and has a nice shopping area from which to stock up on gluten-/dairy-/soy-free Eating Evolved Primal Chocolate, prepared Paleo foods, and Paleo cookbooks. And there are so many other restaurants that are safe for me to eat at that I can't keep up, including Hawthorne and Corbett Fish Houses, Brooklyn House Restaurant, and one of my all-time favorite restaurants, Andina, a Peruvian restaurant in the Pearl District. Andina is not 100 percent gluten free but offers an extensive gluten-free menu, and is very conscientious about preventing cross-contamination.

Another true gem in Portland is the Ground Breaker Brewery, which was the first dedicated gluten-free brewery in the United States. James Neumeister and his team are true artists when it comes to brewing some of the most complex, satisfying, and tasty gluten-free beers. Since I used to like to drink dark ales, my favorite, not surprisingly, is their Dark Ale. An added bonus of visiting Ground Breaker is that they now have a 100 percent gluten-free gastropub, with the kitchen run by Chef Neil Davidson, formerly of Thomas Keller's, The French Laundry, and Ad Hoc. The food and the 100 percent gluten-free beer are hands-down amazingly great. If I didn't live near Portland, I would fly in just to eat at the Ground Breaker. Thankfully, I'm only a short drive away. Whew.

Needless to say, we have access to an astounding array of wonderful foods in this part of the country. But I still panicked initially when I learned I had to go gluten free. My perception of what food was and how much I actually needed to be healthy was skewed. I thought if I did not have access to all of the food products I'd eaten in my previous life, I was certainly going to starve to death. But nothing could be further from the truth. I frequently tell people that I could easily eat strictly from the meat and produce section of my local co-op all year long and never have to eat the same thing twice, unless I wanted to.

Most Americans get into the bad habit of literally eating twenty foods, in some form, over and over, day in and day out. I encourage people to expand their food choices to include fruits and vegetables they have never tried before and to learn how to prepare and eat them. A community sourced agriculture (CSA) box is a great way to step out of your food comfort zone and expose yourself to new fruits and vegetables. CSA boxes forced me to learn about celeriac root, sunchokes, yacón, and various squashes and other tubers. Yum.

The definition of a food desert is "an urban or rural area in which it is difficult to buy affordable or good-quality fresh food." It's safe to say that I do not live in a food desert, but I respectfully recognize that they do exist in America, and I strongly feel they should be illegal. How can we expect people to be healthy and motivated if all they have access to is garbage "food" they can buy at the "food mart" connected to a gas station? Only gas should be bought at a gas station, not "food." This is not food—it is junk that provides no nutritional benefit to the people that eat it. No wonder people are overweight. They are not overweight because they have no self-control. They are overweight because they are starving. All of that extra weight is not because they eat so much good food and therefore pack on a hundred (or two or three hundred) extra pounds. It's because their guts are damaged for any number of reasons, they are eating nutrient-deficient crap "food," and their bodies are storing fat as cheap but nearly useless energy. Once we give people nutrient-dense foods to eat, their intestines heal, they absorb nutrients appropriately, and they tend to come back to their ideal weight. There will always be outliers—the people who have a hard time losing or gaining weight. They have other metabolic and physical issues that need to be addressed, but once these issues are addressed, they will also gain or lose weight as appropriate. This is not rocket science. I believe we can effect a profound shift in the health of our country just by helping people get less of their food from the back of a semi-truck and more of it from the back of a pickup truck.

It's Not a Religion, But It Is Big Business

Wheat is a huge part of our economy. It is one of the United States' and Canada's main export crops. Wheat and other grains are not just considered food; they are commodities traded on Wall Street. Wheat's dominance has also been virtually unchallenged throughout history. I am sure that if someone did raise the alarm about wheat in the past, they may have been killed for heresy. The powerful wheat industry until recently was located in a town in Colorado, but moved its headquarters to Washington D.C., "to combat all of the negative attention wheat is getting in the media." Certainly, the fact that Americans and Canadians are getting educated about the inherent dangers of eating wheat isn't helping the wheat industry's bottom line. By 2013, as noted by the NPD group, a leading global information company, a full 30 percent, or almost one in every three Americans and Canadians, had adopted some form of a gluten-free diet, and this number is expected to increase over the next several years.

Several friends and folks in the general population report to me, though, that their doctors won't test them for celiac disease because they "don't believe in it"—to which I have to incredulously respond, "It's not a religion." We've known about it since the days of the Aretaeus of Cappadocia. *Koiliakos,* aka *the Cœliac Affection,* aka celiac disease is not new and is certainly not a religion, but an actual medical issue. Just because we in America still don't have one single medical textbook on celiac disease does not mean it doesn't exist—it just means it continues to get ignored by the Western medical establishment.

When I talk about celiac disease being a health, social, economic, and political issue, I am not kidding. This is a huge deal. Not just because celiac disease is the largest untapped market in the world. And who might be privy to this fact? The celiac specialists worldwide, for sure. The pharmaceutical companies are certainly aware of celiac disease. The food industry is certainly rolling in the gluten-free dough/money, as evidenced by the sheer number of people who are at least interested in or already on a gluten-free diet. One-third of the North American population is a heck of a lot more than the reported 1 percent of people who are estimated to actually have celiac disease. And as we know, most of the people with actual celiac disease haven't even been diagnosed yet.

How can this all be? Is it really a fad? My favorite is when specialists or practitioners downplay the gluten-free diet for people that haven't been "officially diagnosed with a biopsy" and are therefore not a "true," biopsy-confirmed celiac. The nerve of these people to recognize that they feel better on a gluten-free diet! It must be the "placebo effect." Rubbish. Certain specialists get very upset when people take control of their own health and decisions regarding food and potentially getting better. We have been told by our health-care providers to focus on "diet and exercise" if we want to get healthy. What exactly does that mean? I ate a pretty "healthy" diet by anyone's standards, and I exercised, but my "everything in moderation" lifestyle was the cause of my multi-system organ failure.

My idea of a "healthy" diet then and now is completely different. I had to unlearn, relearn, and continually educate myself on how to truly eat healthy. Both of the tests that were run on me for celiac disease were negative. If I had listened to my doctor, I would have died. She knows that, and so do I. I never had an initial endoscopy because by the time I saw a gastroenterologist, I had already been on a gluten-free diet for several months and was much improved. The gastroenterologist and I agreed that an endoscopy was not necessary, and I certainly knew I was not going on a "gluten challenge" to "prove" I had villous atrophy, to myself, to the doctor, or to anyone else. So, even though I am a homozygous HLA-DQ2.5 who presented with digestive and neurological symptoms, along with very obvious dermatitis herpetiformis—all of which resolved or improved markedly on a strict gluten-free diet—I still am unable to get a diagnosis of celiac disease from the doctors I originally saw. And I don't care.

As we discussed, right around the year 1952, money for research on celiac disease in the U.S. went away. Medical schools stopped teaching about celiac disease in American medical schools. I can find the exact same paragraph in medical textbooks from 1950 and ones written in 2008. Nothing changed. Celiac disease was placed in a time capsule that was never opened in the United States until Dr. Alessio Fasano wrote his landmark paper in 1996 entitled "Where have all the American celiacs gone?"

It was another eight years, in 2004, before the NIH convened a group to determine the best course of action to shed light on the issue of celiac disease in the U.S. They had an opportunity to initiate and implement a mass screening of all Americans, and to educate the public and health care providers all over the country, and they opted to do neither of those things. Even though celiac disease meets the WHO criteria for a mass screening, the testing was not initiated. It was determined that it wasn't "cost effective."

It wasn't until I attended a conference on celiac disease in Chicago sponsored by the American Gastroenterological Association (AGA) in 2009 that I even saw a brochure for the NIH's 2004 Consensus Development Conference on Celiac Disease. There were full boxes of them on the floor at the check-in table. By the looks of it, I imagine that all of the five thousand or so brochures that the NIH had printed were right there in those boxes on the floor. I took two or three of them, but I now realized I should have taken more. They will probably be collector's items in the next few years.

Anyway, as I began my immersion into the subterranean world of gluten intolerance and celiac disease, one of my worldwide web nets caught the NIH's report on the 2004 meeting. It was on this webpage that I learned of this meeting between celiac specialists and other leaders in the celiac world, including representatives of the Celiac Disease Foundation (CDF), the Celiac Sprue Association (CSA), the Gluten Intolerance Group of North America (GIG), and other groups. These specialists, and others with a vested interest in the future of celiac disease, met with the NIH from June 28 to 30 to determine the best strategy to address the "negligence" in looking for and diagnosing celiac disease over the previous several decades in America and to produce a "consensus statement" on celiac disease.

The first paragraph of the conclusion of this consensus statement noted that celiac disease had been "greatly under-diagnosed" and that "heightened awareness... and education of physicians, registered dietitians and other health-care providers is needed." It was also during this meeting that, in light of the "negligence" in acknowledging celiac disease for so long, a "mass screening" for celiac disease in the United States was proposed.

But most of the recommendations that came out of the meeting were never acted on. Education of health-care providers never happened, since most doctors still refer to celiac as a fad and refuse to test patients. There was also a call for the formation of a federation of celiac societies, interest groups, and individuals with celiac disease, but this never happened either. And the idea for a mass screening was ultimately shot down. As noted in the consensus statement: "At this time, there are insufficient data to recommend screening of the general population for celiac disease."

Seriously? You have an opportunity to find millions of people in the United States who are suffering unnecessarily with celiac disease, something that is curable with a diet change, and you opt not to? What possible defense is there for this ruling? Celiac disease meets *all* of the World Health Organization's criteria for a mass screening, which are that:

1. Early clinical detection is difficult.
2. The condition is common.
3. Screening tests are highly sensitive and specific.
4. Effective treatment is available.
5. Untreated disease can lead to complications.

Even if you considered the last two requirements alone, the case for a mass screening is compelling. The "effective treatment" for celiac is a gluten-free diet, and complications are all too often too numerous to count (TNTC), whether individually or collectively, leading to enormously high health-care costs. Multiple worldwide studies have proven that the morbidity (sickness) and mortality (death) rates for undiagnosed celiac patients are exponentially higher than in the constantly referenced "normal" population.

An interesting side note: the mass education of health-care providers recommended during the 2004 meeting was to be led by the National Institute of Diabetes and Digestive and Kidney Disease (NIDDK), in association with the Centers of Disease Control and Prevention (CDC). When I went to the CDC's website, in the A-to-Z listing of diseases, celiac disease was not even there. I called the CDC several times to find out why. One of the women who answered the phone actually asked me if I could spell "celiac" for her. Eventually, I reached someone who explained that celiac disease only comes under the auspices of the NIH. Interesting, since that is *not* what the consensus states.

On the bright side, I learn amazing concepts and meet some of the best people at these conferences. What I remember foremost about the 2009 AGA* conference is that my bladder was still so inflamed that for every tiny cup of hotel coffee I drank, I had to excuse myself and go to the bathroom. The other thought I had at this conference was that I would have loved to present my own topic, "Realities of Celiac Disease: Symptoms, Barriers to Diagnosis, and Living Gluten Free, a Nurse's Perspective." Lacking that opportunity, though, I focused on expanding my outlook, in line with the title of the conference, "Celiac Disease: Broadening Horizons."

But as the conference progressed, I began to understand how celiac disease was being commoditized and funneled through a very narrow, dark pathway leading to… where? Despite compelling questions and answers from every corner, I also became cognizant of a carefully scripted agenda—and even patent bullying—that was being carried out in the company of preeminent world scientists, doctors, and other practitioners at the conference. I had gone seeking answers from the premiere world experts in celiac disease and I left with many more tough questions that I would have to answer for myself over the next several years.

In 2009, I also attended my first Celiac Disease Foundation Expo. I was excited to be part of a community of celiac people, to check out new products, and to hear experts speak about celiac disease. I reconnected with several people, including Anne Roland-Lee, and had the absolute pleasure of hearing her share her own story with a group of registered dietitians. It was during this talk that I learned that Anne's son had stopped growing at one point. He was tested for everything under the sun but had come up negative. Anne suggested, since she worked at the Columbia Celiac Disease Center, that perhaps it would have been a good idea for her son to be tested for celiac disease. And he came up positive on his testing. After a bit of time passed, Anne realized he had to have gotten his genes for celiac from one of his parents, so she was tested for celiac disease too, and came back positive. She worked at the Columbia Celiac Disease Center, where she was employed as the expert celiac disease Registered Dietitian, but she had never thought to get herself or her family screened for celiac disease. Anne is one of my personal and professional idols, and a wealth of knowledge and wisdom. She is now a PhD RD, so she's Dr. Anne Lee (I am so proud of Anne!) and works for Schar USA, a company that provides gluten-free products and education.

We were privileged to have several doctors and experts fly in from the East Coast on tight schedules to present at the expo. What I most remember of those presentations is the following—an example of the narrow, dark pathway down which it seemed some people wanted to take celiac disease... The first few expert speakers told the large group of people with celiac disease how important it was to maintain a 100 percent gluten-free diet. They repeated how even a breadcrumb could cause damage. They talked about refractory celiac disease and how at that point, there is damage done that a gluten-free diet can't heal and people develop lymphoma, which is typically fatal. All of these facts are true and pretty uncontroversial.

But what happened next made my head spin. A doctor who works for a pharmaceutical company stood at the podium and made an impassioned plea for biopsy-proven celiac patients to consider being part of a study that would involve taking them off a gluten-free diet, and having them eat a fair amount of gluten every day. And this would be a double-blind test, so neither the researchers nor the participants in the study would know if they were being given the pill that might or might not prevent damage from the gluten they were now consuming, or if they were being given the placebo, which for very obvious reasons, was not going to help in any way.

I looked around and I could tell there were other nurses in the audience because our brows were furrowed, our mouths were agape, and our heads were shaking. One of the laws or tenets of doing a research study is that you must not cause harm to the subjects who agree to be a part of your study. But here was a very clear example of very real harm potentially occurring. They were suggesting that biopsy-proven celiac patients go off a gluten-free diet, consume gluten, and take either a pill that might or not work or a placebo pill that absolutely *wasn't* going to work.

I then looked around the conference room and realized much of the rest of the crowd were like sheep coming to slaughter. They wanted desperately to believe in the doctors, the celiac experts. Some of them had already been damaged by gluten to the extent that they were walking only with the aid of walkers, canes, or crutches. Some of them had those glazed-over eyes that occur when someone has been brainwashed. These are the vulnerable population that should never be exploited, but here, right before my very eyes, that exact thing was occurring. These experts were soliciting for people to donate their lives, their bodies, and their tenuous health to "science." At one of the Columbia University Celiac Disease Conferences, one of the celiac specialist doctors from Europe spoke up and said, "I don't know how you are able to do these research studies here. In Europe, they are considered unethical."

Dr. Peter Green responded, "Oh, we can do them here. If I ask my patients to participate in a study, they do it."

Is that not only unethical in so many bad and evil ways, but also amoral? It slowly sank through my still-clearing gluten addle-brained skull that the reason the 2004 NIH Consensus Statement on Celiac Disease did not recommend a mass screening despite meeting all of the WHO criteria was because for ten years now, they had been working feverishly to develop, as they now refer to it, a Non-Dietary Treatment Plan for Celiac Disease—a pill, a vaccine, a DNA manipulator, hookworms, or some other novel approach to "treat" what is simply a diet-change-only disease—take the gluten out and people get better. What they don't tell the public is that even if they do come up with a pill or a non-dietary treatment plan for celiac disease, you still have to be on a 100 percent gluten-free diet. The pill is "just in case." Just in case what? Just in case you are fed gluten at a Columbia University Center conference on developing a non-dietary treatment plan for celiac disease?

Remember, this is the largest untapped market in the world. Sample studies have been done worldwide to determine the prevalence of celiac disease. One study that almost flew under my radar was presented at one of the non-dietary treatment plan conferences held at Columbia University. This study had been done by Dr. Rubio Tapas and a team of researchers. It was published in 2006, though I didn't learn about it until a few years later. The study was done in Mexico City using only the anti-tissue transglutaminase 2 (tTG2) component of the celiac testing. What this test clearly showed was that celiac disease exists in this population, even using just one of the actual tests available, at a rate of 1 in 33 for women and 1 in 40 for men. This is much higher than the stated prevalence rate of 1 in 100! Is anyone telling the Hispanic population that they may be at a significantly higher risk for developing celiac disease?!

If you think about it at all, this just makes sense. The American continents, and therefore the Native peoples on both of these continents, from the top to the bottom, were not exposed to grains until less than 500 years ago when these continents were invaded by Europeans, including Christopher Columbus, who brought not only smallpox but also grains. Grains were not indigenous to these continents. There was no wheat, barley, rye, or oats in the Americas. If the Native people grew anything, depending on where they lived, it was corn, squash, and tubers. And even if there were grains, the native peoples had more than enough food to eat and did not need to grow a labor-intensive crop that was poorly digested even by the Mesopotamians who knew that without soaking and fermenting those grains, they would make people sick. The soaking and fermenting of the grains causes the long-chain amino acids to be broken down into smaller amino acids, making the proteins potentially less toxic. I love when people say that "we" have been eating grains for 10,000 years, so those grains have to be good for us, right? Unless your people come from the area of the Fertile Crescent, your people have not been eating grains for ten thousand years.

I gave a talk to some of the local Native American tribal members a few years back. I was enormously excited to finally have an inroad into the Native population. If there is one group for which I have been enthusiastically voicing my desire for a mass screening for celiac disease, it is this population. Way back in 2008, I wrote a blog post that specifically asked, "Why isn't there one study in the whole country on the incidence of celiac disease in the Native American population?" When I do a Google search to see if there are any current studies available on this topic, my blog post is still the number-one result. A PubMed search for "Native Americans Celiac Disease" shows no related research articles either. None.

Most of the people who attended my class that day were older and had diabetes or other chronic health issues. They listened raptly to what I had to say, and asked very relevant questions. I talked about the Paleo diet and hunter-gatherer cultures. I point-blank suggested that their health issues were potentially related to the food they were eating. They smiled and nodded, agreeing wholeheartedly.

Near the end of the talk, though, one woman spoke up. "I would love to eat good food," she said, "but I am poor. The only food we have access to really is subsidized food, which is wheat, grains, corn, milk, and processed cheese. We truly cannot afford to eat well."

I felt like a complete and total schmuck, in an educated, entitled-white-nurse kind of way. I had let my passion for the information override the assessment of the group I was speaking to. Thankfully, I have since learned of several tribes making internal efforts nationwide to strongly encourage the return to more native diets—basically, what the native people ate before white people, small pox, and grains, none of which are indigenous to these continents, invaded North and South Americas.

How we provide calories to the poor and vulnerable people in this country in the form of nutrient-deficient, subsidized and processed foods is morally reprehensible. We all understand that we can't turn back the clocks and eat entirely a hunter-gatherer or strictly native diet, but a move in that direction would be medically, socially, and culturally advantageous. And nothing would make me happier than to help with a study to find out the prevalence of celiac disease in the Native population and work for the rest of my days to find ways to restore health and well-being to the Native Peoples of North and South America.

If a person is diagnosed with celiac disease in Italy, they are automatically set up with follow-up appointments, they have extra paid days from work for these appointments and to shop for gluten-free foods, and they are sent a box of gluten-free food, regardless of where they are in the world, for free every month. The U.K. has a publicly and privately funded Coeliac Society. Patients in the U.K. are given a prescription to take to the pharmacy, and the pharmacists help them pick out gluten-free foods. Italy, the U.K., and most other industrialized countries have some form of universal health care. Those governments know it is much cheaper to feed people gluten free than it is to deal with the potential medical sequelae (complications and further conditions) that occur when people are not completely gluten free.

"Let food be thy medicine and let thy medicine be thy food", as Hippocrates famously stated. So food is medicine and is treated as such by many universal health-care systems around the world. How progressive is that? It's totally progressive, and it just makes sense. But in the United States, where as we discussed, it takes an average of nine to fifteen years to get diagnosed (if ever), many people die without ever knowing it was celiac disease, an easily treatable condition, that killed them. It is for this and many other reasons that I work diligently for universal health care for the United States. I am talking about basic medical care, not giving everyone a new Mercedes every year. This is basic medical care like every other industrialized nation in the world has, but we Americans are so afraid of having access to medical care, and the insurance, medical, and pharmaceutical industries are so happy-drunk on their profits that they aren't giving up the smoke and mirrors. Why in heaven's name would the current dictators of our "health-care" system want anything to change? They'd rather keep people sick and order expensive tests than to test those people for celiac disease and teach them how to get better using real, whole foods.

It is horrifying every time a family has some catastrophic medical condition, and they and their communities have to hold car washes, bake sales, and fundraisers just to stay above water. All too often, these families face medical bankruptcy through no fault of their own. Many of these families even have health insurance, but find themselves in dire straits due to the sheer avalanche of medical bills. If you are a nurse, doctor, or medical professional of any kind, please consider joining Physicians for a National Health Plan, Health Care For All, or another local grassroots group that is actively working toward single-payer health care. Countries with universal health care are actively looking for people with celiac disease, because the sooner people get diagnosed correctly, the less money they cost the system.

Don't be afraid of health care for all. I have been a nurse for well over twenty years, and I, for one, am ashamed and appalled we are having these conversations about basic health care in 2015. Seriously? Honestly, it *is* 2015, right?

Get. Everyone. Tested.

My entire life has prepared me for what my calling is now. Sort of like I'm on a mission from God, similar to, but also significantly different from the Blues Brothers. I wear sunglasses only on sunny days. So far, I do not have entities chasing me down to do me harm. Yet.

Still, every day, to some poor soul, I have to apologize for the medical care they did or did not receive. I have to say something like, "I am sorry that happened to you. You should not have had to go through all of that for one/ten/twenty/thirty years to only to find out you had celiac disease all along, but you were just never tested. I am sorry." Too many people tell me of their epic efforts to obtain reliable medical advice and care only to be told they are making up their symptoms, there is nothing wrong with them, or they are hypochondriacs. As a crusty, seasoned emergency nurse, I fully realize that some of them very well may be making up their symptoms and complaints. But the vast majority, we are too slowly finding out, are actually gluten intolerant or meet the current criteria for a celiac disease diagnosis. Why is it taking so long to identify these poor, suffering souls who pay good money for what they assume is good medical care but get few if any answers, sometimes for years, about why they have these mystifying symptoms that persist, worsen, segue into other maladies and years of misery, and even end in dementia, immobility, or early death?

This book is written for those of you still suffering. As a nurse, not being able to self-diagnose my plethora of seemingly incongruent gastric, neurological, and skin symptoms was maddening. I completely understand the frustration people feel when they tell me they are sick but that no one knows what is wrong with them or how they can get better. They see doctor after doctor but never seem to get to the bottom of their illness or symptoms. Many times their lab work looks great on paper, or they have what appear to be slight bumps in some of their levels that are dismissed as nothing. But these people suffer and die without knowing that the root cause of their symptoms is actually the food they have been eating their entire lives, despite their thinking they were consuming the "right" foods according to all mainstream recommendations.

Those of you who have lost friends or family members to mystery diseases, take heart. If your family members are getting sick and dying, sometimes very young, then it would be a very important piece of the puzzle to identify whether you are at risk of gluten intolerance or celiac disease. And even if your family seems to have longevity and health right up to the end, grains may still be affecting your family's health in ways we are just now beginning to understand.

Illnesses that cause morbidity and mortality are very important to identify and act upon, especially if the cause can be identified, removed, or treated. The WHO refers to this as "burden of disease" (BOD) and they strive to lessen BOD because of the immense financial and social toll that disease can take on a population of people. Unfortunately, those of us who live in the United States of America have to try to function in a for-profit health care society that reaps financial benefit only when we the people *are* sick. The system bills us for tests, medications, appointments, procedures, and surgeries that never really seem to fix the underlying problem. Our medical providers are good at prescribing medications for symptoms but not so great at diagnosing the root cause of all of those accumulating symptoms.

But there is also an economic incentive—at least for insurers—to get more people tested for celiac disease. The insurance industry knows that less money is spent on people the sooner they are diagnosed, according to a 2008 article by Peter Green, MD, et al in the *Journal of Insurance Medicine* entitled "Economic benefits of increased diagnosis of celiac disease in a national managed care population in the United States." As a matter of fact, if an insurance company denies payment for celiac testing, I pull out this study, call the insurance company and use it to encourage them to reverse their denial.

With my strong background in emergency, trauma, and critical care, I am telling you, without any doubt, that your health is all about the food you eat. I had no idea that the wounds we were trying to heal would never heal if the patient was malnourished, or stuck on the Standard American Diet (aka SAD), which is the case if the grains we eat every day have damaged the lining of the small intestines. Additionally, if the intestines, otherwise known as your guts, are damaged, so is your immune system. This is particularly scary given that we now live in a world in which the antibiotics we have relied on for decades are no longer effective against certain bacteria—so-called "superbugs," which include *Neisseria gonorrhoeae,* Carbapenem-resistant Enterobacteriaceae (CRE), and *Clostridium difficile.* With 70 to 90 percent of our immune system in our guts, it is imperative that we all work as diligently as possible to heal our guts, and thereby our immune systems. If you have what is commonly known as "leaky gut" or increased permeability of your intestinal wall, then your number one goal in life needs to be to heal that leaky gut. The reality is, if you have a leaky gut, you also have a leaky blood-brain barrier, leaky blood vessels, leaky lungs, and leaky skin. Your integumentary system is failing and allowing antigens, undigested food particles, yeast, viruses, and bacteria into your bloodstream. The result is that our immune systems are so inflamed and malfunctioning that we end up with multiple allergies and intolerances to substances and foods that make no sense.

For all of you who just assume you are doomed to develop cancer, dementia, arthritis, Alzheimer's, or any other genetic or familial disease or early death, there is HOPE. Everything you think you know is rubbish. Finding this out the hard way is like a slap in the face. It is a paradigm shift from what you thought you knew to a new reality. You have been duped, but there is potentially an easy remedy for what ails our families and our communities. It all boils down to the food you eat. The sad truth is that we as a country have been duped into believing wheat and grains are good, healthy and nutritious, providing necessary daily vitamins and minerals. Nothing could be further from the truth.

Hospitals are notorious for serving the most unhealthy, nutrient-deficient, dead foods ever. This is one of the main reasons I no longer work as a nurse in hospitals. Number one, I can't eat the food, since the risk of cross-contamination is enormous, and number two, I would be very vocal about getting the patients, the nurses, the doctors, the cleaning staff, and the administrators all tested correctly for celiac disease. One of my doctor friends laughingly told me I would get fired within ten minutes of showing up for my shift. I laughed too, knowing he was ribbing me, but that what he said was also the truth.

I have given well over 1,300 lectures on over seventy-five topics related to gluten intolerance, celiac disease, the gut-brain-skin connection, nutrient-dense foods, emergency preparedness classes for people with food issues, the Paleo diet and lifestyle, the gut microbiome, and most recently, my favorite, fecal microbial transplants. I have presented at formal conferences, local food fairs and expos, universities, doctors' and dentists' offices, neighborhood gatherings, and private family meetings. Never in my wildest dreams as an emergency nurse did I ever imagine looking forward to and enjoying the process of presenting a lecture on anything, let alone the power of food choices. I am having so much fun, and I really love to hear people's stories of regaining their health just by changing their diet.

I have consulted with thousands of patients and their families. I understand the correlative and causal relationships that are so important to medical research and to prove my hypotheses and theories are correct. What I also understand is that everyone is their own science experiment. A study of one. Interestingly, celiac disease is so diverse in its presentation, so all over the board with symptoms and complaints from patient to patient, that doctors complain that it is too complicated to pick out the people to test for celiac disease. For this reason alone, celiac disease should at least be on every patient's differential diagnosis. Let me make it very simple for medical practitioners. Do what some of your forward-thinking colleagues are doing, and test everyone. Yes, everyone. Do your own mass screening of your patients.

My favorite questions to ask doctors are, "How many patients with celiac disease do you have in your practice?" and "How many people have you diagnosed with celiac disease?" One of my other favorite questions to ask them is, "Have you and your family been tested for celiac disease?" This is how change happens more quickly, when doctors and people in the medical field realize that they too are affected. This is how the cultural change from "it's a fad" to "it's a public health crisis" (because it is) happens faster.

My conundrum as a nurse is getting people tested as recommended, since there are some serious issues with the commonly prescribed testing methods for celiac disease. Getting tested for celiac disease can be a murky endeavor. Understand that there is not one simple test available that will rule you in as celiac or as gluten intolerant. This is a problem for patients and practitioners alike. There are several confounding problems with the serum or blood antibody testing that makes it somewhere in the range of 70 percent false negative nationwide. There is lab-to-lab variability, which means you can send blood drawn from the same patient on the same day to two different labs and get different results. Patients can also seroconvert, which means their lab tests can be negative one month, but a few months later, when enough organ damage has occurred, their test will "convert" to positive.

These are some of the reasons you can be ruled IN for celiac disease, but you can never be ruled OUT, even if you are not a carrier of HLA-DQ2 and/or HLA-DQ8, the two genetic alleles that have been determined to be necessary to develop celiac disease proper. If you are a celiac gene carrier, it means you are predisposed to developing celiac disease at any time in your life. If you are a homozygous gene carrier, which means you received a gene from each parent, your risk of developing celiac disease is much higher, or as I like to say, "You are almost guaranteed to develop celiac disease." Finding out you are a gene carrier is not considered to be diagnostic itself, but it can be an important part of the puzzle. Many labs are only testing for these two genes associated with celiac disease, but scientists all over the world are looking at least thirty-nine more genes, and "possibly thousands" of other ones.

There are reasons that some researchers consider the blood antibody test to be "highly sensitive and specific," but it's not. If it is approached from the front side, you find that roughly 1 percent of "white" people (those presumed to have their ethnicity rooted somewhere in Europe) actually have a positive blood antibody test. But the only way a blood antibody test comes back positive is if you *already* have significant damage to your intestines and your body is mounting an autoimmune response.

Under the current system of diagnosing celiac disease, the patient is then sent to a gastroenterologist for an endoscopy for biopsies of the duodenum to confirm the positive blood test. This is despite the fact that the biopsies are no longer considered the "gold standard" and are more typically referred to as "tarnished bronze" by anyone in the celiac community, except for the one or two practitioners still clinging to their endoscopes. But many people still undergo an endoscopy for biopsy to become a "biopsy-proven" celiac. They clutch their biopsy-proven diagnosis as proof of their elite status as a REAL celiac; everyone else is either faking it or just jumping on the gluten-free bandwagon and trying to make it harder for the REAL celiac patients to eat safely. Meanwhile, the people whose tests are "negative" are told to go ahead and eat whatever they want, and certainly not to go on a gluten-free diet, because it is very hard/expensive/dangerous/can make you fat.

Within the current medical system, not everyone is or will have the opportunity to get tested, ever. Many Americans don't have health insurance. Some Americans don't have access to health-care practitioners who know anything about celiac disease. In a concerted effort to have all of my RN On Call clients tested for celiac disease, I request that their primary care provider test them every year. One doctor told me that she considered it a disservice to her patients to diagnose celiac disease because the diet was so hard. Really? Do you not diagnose cancer either because the surgery, chemotherapy, and radiation are so hard? Another doctor told me that my patient's diagnoses of early-onset dementia, balance issues, anemia, and osteoporosis didn't meet the criteria for testing for celiac disease. Really? That's just not true. When I stated that was not true, she responded that she only based her decisions on current standard-of-care requirements and that she utilized evidenced-based medicine. Sure, but are you reading any research articles that have come out recently? Like in the last ten years?

A registered dietitian who took one of my classes called me afterward and said she had reviewed several of her hospital inpatients' charts. "You are NOT going to believe what I found!"

she exclaimed to me.

"Oh, go ahead, try me," I said.

"One of my thirty-eight-year-old patients, a mother with four kids who has several autoimmune diagnoses, including debilitating arthritis, is in the hospital more than out, and is on high-dose prednisone and every other medication you can think of... . Well, she was tested for celiac disease six years ago. And her antibody test was positive. But nobody told her she has celiac disease. She has celiac disease, clear as day. The labs were buried in the back of her chart, but they were clearly positive."

Tragically, I believe her. The truth is always more frightening than any fiction you can ever come up with, ever. I encourage people to bring in their lab results for celiac disease so I can review them. Another pair of eyes never hurts, right? People have actually come into my office with what their doctor has said was a negative test for celiac disease. I've looked the paper over and said, "Really, can your doctor actually read? Because it says right here, in English, that this is a positive test for celiac disease." This never ceases to amaze me. If these are the tests that people are having done and they are being read incorrectly, how often is this occurring not just with celiac panels, but with every test?

Here we have issues with accessibility to basic testing, insurance issues, obstacles for ordering the correct tests, correct interpretation of the test results, and general misinformation about what being on a gluten-free diet means to a person and their family. If people genuinely can't afford testing or have been tested almost to death, for everything except for celiac disease, what are their options? Or if they were tested and their tests were negative for celiac disease but they have nothing to lose by going gluten free, shouldn't they be fully supported in their efforts to potentially heal and be symptom free? Who gets to be the judge about someone being gluten free as long as they feel better, have access to up-to-date information and food that is not cross-contaminated, and are preventing themselves from developing some chronic disease for which there is no treatment or cure?

When there is a shooting event in the United States, inevitably someone will call me, especially after the shooter is apprehended and their picture is broadcast, and they will say things like, "Nadine, did you see that picture? That person looks like they have celiac disease. Can't you call someone? Let them know!"

Sure, but not really. Who would I call? The FBI? The CIA? Ask them to test the shooter for celiac disease? In the absence of real proof, it would be difficult to suggest that someone had celiac disease based solely on a grainy photo. But I am quite certain the intestinal mucosa does not miraculously heal upon death, and that the intestinal organ damage would be evident on autopsy. So I did the best thing I could think of at the time. I called the Oregon State Medical Examiner (ME) and asked him to test all dead people with sudden, violent, or drug-related deaths for celiac disease, on autopsy.

The ME's gruff and cranky response was, "You need to talk to a gastroenterologist, not me."

"No, I am talking to the right person," I said. "You are the state medical examiner, correct? You do autopsies on all of the people who died sudden, unexplained, violent deaths, right? I am talking about testing dead people for celiac disease. Dead people are under your auspices for testing, correct?"

He responded loudly, as if I was not listening or too stupid to understand, "You need to talk to a gastroenterologist, not me."

So I called up our local medical examiner, a very nice woman, and asked if it was possible to detect or test for celiac disease on autopsy.

She said, "We certainly can test for it and the intestinal inflammation and damage is detectable on autopsy." She recommended I contact OHSU and suggest they do a research study to determine how much and to what extent undiagnosed celiac disease is showing up in dead people. We as an office have also applied for a grant to run a study, which was "approved but not funded," to do research related to cardiac issues and gluten.

What you have to understand is that while there are common denominators in the gluten intolerance and celiac disease population, there are many more individual case presentations. We are all our own science experiment. We are all a study of one. Become your own science experiment and experiment with your food. First, get yourself and your family tested for celiac disease so you have a baseline. If the test is positive, great, welcome to the club. If it is negative, decide whether you want to pursue further testing, such as the genetic testing, or whether you just want to try the experiment of going gluten free.

But if you already know you are a gene carrier for celiac disease and you have ANY symptoms, please consider going gluten free as soon as possible. Why do people need to be told to wait until they have Marsh IV intestinal damage before they are given the opportunity to improve their health and their lives? This is a quality-of-life issue. Your choices impact all of those around you, including future generations, not just immediately but in the short and long-term. Take gluten 100 percent out of your diet. Not just for a few weeks and no time off during the weekends.

It is frustrating to hear folks say things like, "Sure, I am on a gluten-free diet, but I have my beer every night or every weekend." See if you have more energy, your skin issues improve, you sleep better, and your autoimmune diseases resolve or improve markedly. There is no harm in going on a gluten-free diet, despite what you may have heard. You have nothing to lose except weight, pain, inflammation, irritation, and the list goes on. Plus, you are preventing who knows what health issues down the road. My personal and professional goal is to stay healthy until I die at a ripe and still very plucky old age.

If you think gluten intolerance and celiac disease doesn't affect you, your family and your friends, think again. Gluten intolerance and celiac disease potentially affects everyone and anyone. Rich people. Poor people. White people. Polish people. Angry people. Meek people. Black, brown and tan people. At any age, intrauterine fetuses, newborns, toddlers, teenagers, young adults, adults and seniors. Any ethnicity. With any symptom or no symptoms at all. Hispanic people. Irish people. Aboriginals, Italian people. Chinese people. Jewish people. Native American people. First Nation people. Inuits. Russians. People on every continent worldwide.

When I tell people we are the largest untapped market in the world, I am not kidding.

In order to determine the true prevalence of celiac disease, I would like to suggest the first mass screening for celiac disease: multi-ethnic, no one is excluded, with the possible exception of children under the age of two or three because their immune systems are immature and they tend to have an even higher rate of false negatives—but we can certainly still gene-test these children. Even eight years ago, when I first started getting educated, I was calling for someone, anyone, everyone, to do their own study, mass screening, specific population study—whatever they could get a grant for or self-fund. I have publicly called for such a mass screening at several of the celiac conferences. But in lieu of actually getting to test absolutely everyone, these are the groups I would like to test immediately, if not sooner:

- Developmentally delayed people
- People with Down, Turner, and Williams Syndrome
- The prison population
- Mean, nasty, irritable, grumpy, and angry people
- Women in general, but especially women with fertility issues
- Men in general, but especially men with gas, gastric reflux, anemia and osteopenia/osteoporosis, erectile dysfunction, fertility issues, or autoimmune issues
- People with any mental health conditions such as anxiety, depression, bipolar, schizophrenia, or brain fog
- People in rehab for ANY addiction issue: alcohol, cigarettes, gambling, meth, cocaine, heroin, the QVC channel, etc., etc.
- People with eating disorders
- Children in general
- Children with short stature, learning disabilities, anger issues, developmental issues, vision and hearing issues,

bedwetting, irritability, etc., etc.

- Obese people before they opt for gastric bypass or bariatric surgery
- Elderly people, especially those in memory care units or diagnosed with dementia or "Alzheimer's"
- African Americans
- Native Americans
- Hispanic Americans
- Asian Americans
- Polish Americans (mostly because I am Polish)
- People with red hair (like me)
- People with hazel eyes (like me)
- People with a positive Braly's Sign, first noted in 1953 by Dr. James Braly, which is where the fifth digit/finger is equal to or shorter than the distal joint on the fourth digit. This is a noted association with celiac disease that is not considered diagnostic but points to a potential deficiency during intra uterine development
- People with a longer second toe than their first toe
- Doctors and their families
- Adults
- Anyone diagnosed with ANY autoimmune disease
- Short people
- Tall people
- Overweight people
- Skinny people
- People with blond hair
- People with blue eyes
- People with brown eyes

Okay. In case you haven't figured it out by now, that's my long-winded way of reiterating that I would like EVERYONE tested. I am an equal-opportunity, all-inclusive nurse: Everybody In, Nobody Out. I also want us to challenge some of these deep-rooted beliefs about celiac testing that seem to be difficult to dispel. Not everyone has damage to their intestines. Celiac disease is primarily a neurological disease, even though for years celiac disease has been under the auspices of gastroenterology, which is maybe why the endoscopic biopsy was considered the "gold standard" for too long.

Evidence-based medicine is not meant to be based only on peer-reviewed research, but is supposed to review all of the patient's symptoms and options, and take into account the patient's wishes for treatment. One of my primary beefs about people wielding peer-reviewed research like a club is that not all of this research is held to the same standards. My antenna immediately gets a hit and my radar calls my Bat Phone if a doctor or scientist won't discuss an option or talk about celiac disease because of "evidence-based research." Or if they refuse to discuss any other possibilities other than what their study concludes. Or if they refuse to take into account all of the other research done worldwide that challenges or refutes their results.

Well, let's talk about so-called peer-reviewed, evidence-based medicine and how well it is working out for patients. Let's also talk about the variables and factors that are omitted from various studies. Let's talk about who paid for the studies and who might benefit financially. Let's find out if the doctors and researchers are taking ANY money from pharmaceuticals. Is this being disclosed? Let's talk about all of these issues before anyone starts to be a bully, swinging their peer-reviewed-evidence-based-medicine-spiked bat at your poor head. Wear a helmet. And think critically.

Reader's Guide to Getting Tested and Going Gluten Free

Part 1: Getting Tested

When people say they don't have celiac, disease I ask them, "Really? How do you know?" The typical response is, "I don't really know, but I am fine and I can eat anything I want. Wheat doesn't make me sick." It may be true that they have no symptoms that they recognize. In my previous life, I would have said I had no symptoms either. But the fact was, I had no frame of reference for what "normal" looked and felt like because I had always felt that way. Somewhere in the vicinity of 40 to 60 percent of the newly diagnosed population would say they have no symptoms, even though they have positive blood tests and detectable villous atrophy.

If someone responds, "My doctor tested me for that and I don't have it," my response is always this: "At this point in history, you can be ruled IN for celiac disease, but you can never be ruled OUT." Our testing options are not foolproof, by any stretch of the imagination. When I mention that the auto-antibody test is 70 percent false negative nationwide, people are stunned. I am not even sure why we still do it. You can test negative at one lab, but positive at another with the same blood sample. You can seroconvert, which means that in January you don't have enough damage to your intestines to stimulate the antibodies to have a positive result, but by April you have enough damage to your intestines to have antibodies in your blood that show you "now" have celiac disease.

Plus, the standard auto-antibody tests currently being run in the United States are only testing for the anti-tissue transglutaminase 2 (tTG2), which tests for widespread or intestinal damage. The anti-tissue transglutaminase 3 (tTG3) is specific for dermatitis herpetiformis and other skin and hair issues. The anti-tissue transglutaminase 6 (tTG6) is specific for the neurological components and for gluten ataxia. If the lab you are using doesn't test for tTG6—and most people with celiac disease present with at least one neurological symptom—then they are actively missing most people who would test positive when given the correct test. At this point, Cyrex Labs is the only lab in the United States that offers anti-tissue transglutaminase 2, 3, and 6 testing, along with 21 other antibodies specific to grains (wheat, barley, and rye), on their Array 3 test.

As a nurse, I want celiac testing to be cheaper, easier, and more inclusive. But finding out you are intolerant to wheat or actually celiac by the current standards is no easy feat. One celiac panel or celiac antibody test is insufficient to tell a person they don't have celiac disease, nor whether they will they ever get it. There are so many variables for each person and each family that the options can be overwhelming. Your chances of actually having celiac disease but having the tests come back negative or even "borderline" is still quite high. And the slate of testing options we have now is confusing. When people ask me which test is best for them to order, it is tricky and usually not clear-cut. Do you have insurance? Are you private pay? Who is your doctor? Which lab do they use? If the lab is sent out to another lab, which lab is it? Does your practitioner have access to Cyrex Labs? Do you want to order your own genetic testing through a web-based company? Can your doctor order genetic testing? Is the testing for a child? Are you interested in a stool analysis? Are you interested in a blood test? Saliva? Stool? Does the lab automatically do a Total IgA and IgG test as part of the Celiac Panel or does it need to be ordered separately? Does the person looking at the test results know how to interpret them? I am not a geneticist, but I have geneticists on my speed dial if I can't figure out exactly what the results are on the report.

Hopefully I've drilled into your head the importance of getting tested, but it's clear that the state of celiac testing is less than ideal—unfortunately, there isn't one simple, foolproof test that will rule you in or out for celiac disease. So with that in mind, how do you actually go about it? As a general set of recommendations, here are the tests you should look to get to determine your celiac status:

A serum (blood) test that includes Total IgA and Total IgG, Anti-tTG IgA and Anti-tTG IgG, Anti-EMA, DGP and an AGA

These will need to be ordered by your PCP (this is the test that is potentially 70 percent false negative nationwide) If this test is positive, great, you are in the celiac club—but if it is negative, it doesn't mean much.

Total IgA and Total IgG; If you are IgA deficient, then the rest of the test will most likely be negative because you are unable to mount an immune response, and other testing will need to be pursued. A significant number of people who prove to be celiac are noted to be IgA deficient on their initial test. These people need additional testing, including, but not limited to a duodenal biopsy by a competent endoscopist.

Anti-tTG IgA and Anti-tTG IgG: Anti-Tissue Transglutaminase Immunoglobulin A (IgA) and Anti-Tissue Transglutaminase Immunoglobulin (IgG)

Anti-EMA: Anti-Endomysial Antibodies IgA and IgG

DGP: Deamidated Antigliadin Peptide

AGA: Anti-Gliadin Antibody. Several labs have removed this test from the celiac panel because it is not considered sensitive or specific for celiac disease. Dr. Hadjivassiliou considers the AGA to be an excellent biomarker, as do I, if not specifically for celiac disease, then for gluten intolerance. If you are lucky enough to have a lab that still runs this as part of their celiac panel, it can provide a valuable piece of the diagnostic puzzle.

Cyrex Labs Array 3

This will also need to be ordered by your PCP. Array 3 includes the Tissue Transglutaminase 2, 3, and 6 tests. Although the serum blood testing (as noted above) includes the anti-tissue transglutaminase 2, it does not include the anti-tissue transglutaminase 3 test, which indicates skin damage, or the anti-tissue transglutaminase 6 test, which indicates neurological damage. Cyrex is the only lab that is currently providing this level of testing, and not every practitioner has access to this lab yet, which is unfortunate.

Celiac gene or DNA testing for HLA-DQ2 and/or DQ8.

This can be ordered by your PCP, or can be self-ordered from several reputable companies. Genetic testing can be very helpful, depending on which lab you choose, and as long as you understand that DNA is just part of the puzzle. Being an HLA-DQ2 and/or DQ8 gene carrier predisposes a person to celiac disease, but is not considered diagnostic. Having said that, if you are a carrier of genes associated with celiac disease and you are eating wheat, barley, rye and oats you are at risk for developing celiac disease. When the only testing available to people was the self-ordered genetic testing through Kimball Genetics, we utilized that testing. And when those tests came back positive for HLA-DQ2 and/or HLA-DQ8 and they had any of the 300-plus symptoms related to celiac disease, my recommendation to them was to get a celiac disease blood test and then consider going gluten free, whether the test was positive or negative.

Is the DNA test accurate? Yes, whether you are on a gluten-free diet or not. In fact, it is the only test you can do once you are on a gluten-free diet that will be accurate, because your genes won't change. There are a few caveats, depending on which lab you choose. The other most important fact to remember is that there are many more genes involved in celiac disease, along with the epigenetic factors or environmental triggers that turn these genes on and off. So why do you need to be genetically tested if it's not diagnostic? A genetic test can be a great indicator of the family members at greatest risk for developing celiac disease, and it can be helpful in cementing a diagnosis of celiac disease even in case of a negative blood test or intestinal biopsy, neither of which are highly accurate for many reasons.

My current favorite company to order genetic testing is from Glutenpro, which is in headquartered in Toronto, Canada. This company runs the test for celiac genetics and the charge is under $200 Canadian, which is very reasonable for genetic testing. Note that you can't pay with a check because of 9/11; it has to be with a credit card. If you go this route for testing, call Glutenpro or have them call you when they receive your sample kit to get your credit card information so it isn't on the paperwork. You can also order their E-Z Gluten test kits, which test food and drinks for gluten to less than 10 ppm, along with the elusive-in-the-United States BioCard for $55. You can access this information at www.glutenpro.com.

Enterolab also offers genetic testing. One benefit of EnteroLab's DNA test is that they also test for the gluten sensitivity genes, which no other lab is currently providing. However, keep in mind that Enterolab's testing for HLA-DQ2 and DQ8 includes the beta subunit of DQ2 but not the alpha subunit. I have had a few people test positive only for the HLA-DQ2 alpha subunit when using other genetic testing labs.

Stool analysis for anti-gliadin antibodies and fat malabsorption.

This is offered by EnteroLab and can be self-ordered from www.enterolab.com. Originally, I believed some of the scuttle on the web that EnteroLab was a scam. I hadn't had any experience with them, and being a naturally skeptical person, I was leery. Then people started to bring me self-ordered test results, and I was impressed by the information on their reports; particularly invaluable is the fat-malabsorption portion of the testing. Keep in mind this is how the children in the 1920s, '30s, '40s, and into the '50s were diagnosed with celiac disease, when they would present with steatorrhea or fatty foul smelling stools. Also note that the Enterolab results are worth waiting for, but it can take five to six weeks to get them back.

Baseline and follow-up lab testing.

This should always be done on a newly diagnosed celiac patient to establish a baseline for deficiencies and to help identify organs that are damaged. At the very least, the following labs are necessary in order to establish a baseline:

- Complete blood count (CBC)
- Complete metabolic panel (CMP)
- Vitamin D3 level
- Vitamin B12 level
- Magnesium RBC level (*not* a serum level)
- Thyroid panel
- Bone density test
- Lipid panel

Finally, keep in mind that a person has to be eating gluten to have any of the celiac antibody testing done. If a person has decided to go on a gluten-free diet before getting any of the antibody testing, then that person can always get a genetic test done, but I never, ever recommend someone go back to eating any amount of gluten for any amount of time in order to "prove" they have celiac disease, especially if they had symptoms that resolved on a gluten-free diet. There are way too many serious variables, complications, and other factors that make this route inaccurate and potentially dangerous.

If I could create a perfect test, it would be quick, easy, cheap and available to everyone. Several years ago, I came across a point of care test kit called BioCard that is manufactured in Finland. This is a home test kit for the anti-tissue transglutaminase 2 IgA antibody, aka the anti-tTg2. I got on my computer, ordered up a case of the test kits, and paid several hundred dollars with my Visa. My plan was to offer the test kits to people at cost so people could have access to something along with the genetic testing. Unfortunately, the following morning I received an email from the company in Finland notifying me that they would be happy to bill me and send the test kits, but they kindly advised me that the kits would be confiscated by the FDA because they were not approved for use in the United States.

But these same test kits are available as over-the-counter test kits in pharmacies all across Canada and in many other countries. People in other countries can literally say to themselves, "Gee, I think I would like to test myself for celiac disease today," or "How well am I doing on my gluten-free diet?" then go to a pharmacy, buy a test kit for about $50, and go home and test themselves with a simple finger-poke blood sample. This is referred to as point of care testing, or POCT. It's similar to a home pregnancy test, but for celiac disease. How cool is that? What a novel idea! I later learned that even though these kits are still not available in the U.S., you can order them online through Canada and should be okay to order enough for "a family."

I am currently trying to get a lab to perform all of the testing that I think is helpful in quickly and accurately identifying celiac patients. I have sent at least two letters to Theranos offering my assistance in developing cheap, easy, and accurate testing for gluten intolerance and celiac disease. So far, Theranos has not jumped on my offer. I am anticipating a phone call from Elizabeth Holmes of Theranos any day now.

What About the Biopsy?

The intestinal biopsy is no longer considered the "gold standard" by many celiac specialists, as it is fraught with errors. The standard number of intestinal samples to be taken is a minimum of six, but rarely is this standard of care met. It has been confirmed in multiple studies that the more samples that are taken from different areas of the intestines, the more likely it is that the test will reveal areas of villous atrophy and blunting, and the more likely a diagnosis of celiac disease will be made. The intestinal damage from celiac disease can be patchy, so taking anything fewer than six samples from a twenty-to-thirty-foot-long gastrointestinal tract is less than optimal.

The samples also have to be prepared properly and applied to the slide in the correct orientation. Whoever is reading the tissue samples has to know what they are looking for with Marsh I, II, III or IV damage. Tragically, I have been privy to too many cases where patients were told they had intestinal damage but it wasn't Marsh IV yet, so they didn't need to go on a gluten-free diet yet. Whoa. Why in the bloody hell would you wait until you had MORE organ damage before you diagnosed celiac disease? Marsh I damage is sufficient to diagnose along with signs and symptoms, gene carrier status, and perhaps a positive antibody test.

It would have been a different experience in the emergency department if we had determined that patients were having myocardial infarctions aka heart attacks via blood tests and procedures, but then telling them wasn't enough damage YET, so go home and keep doing what you are doing, here is a prescription for pain medication and a little something for that nausea until you have MORE of a heart attack and THEN we will see about treating you with medications and procedures and surgery. We all know that time is heart muscle or brain tissue in the instance of a stroke, so we have strict standards of care that help ensure that patients at risk for tissue damage and therefore death are seen emergently, diagnosed appropriately, and treated within tight time parameters. Why is it so hard to understand that the people with villous atrophy also have massive organ damage that, if they are allowed to continue eating gluten, could be irreversible? This condition is called refractory celiac disease. It is a T-cell lymphoma, and while there are chemotherapy treatments, they are certainly not a cure. This is a situation where the damage is done and can't be undone, even on a 100 percent gluten-free diet.

I have been in the endoscopy suite during biopsies with clients who have a positive blood test. It was during one particular biopsy procedure that the endoscopist went two inches into the duodenum, took two samples, and declared that my patient with a positive blood test did not have celiac disease. This incorrect information delayed my patient going on a gluten-free diet for another two years, during which time she became sicker and more debilitated. Her excuse for not going on a gluten-free diet was that "the doctor said I don't have celiac disease because my biopsy was negative." According to the University of Chicago Celiac Disease Center, if you have a positive anti-tTG2 and anti-EMA (endomysial antibodies), then you have gut damage. Intestinal damage is the only way to trigger those two tests to be positive.

The question begs to be answered: if this is the case, do people really need to have a biopsy at all, especially considering it is no longer considered the gold standard but only the tarnished bronze? As we have come to realize that more people have neurological damage instead of intestinal damage and symptoms, then is the endoscopy necessary other than in cases where the serum/blood antibody test is negative but there is still suspicion of intestinal damage based on symptoms, malnutrition, and/or family history?

Some people still want the confirmation of intestinal damage before they agree to a diagnosis of celiac disease and a lifelong 100 percent gluten free lifestyle change, which is fine. But unfortunately, I have clients, family, and friends who are gene carriers for either HLA-DQ2 or DQ8, have a positive celiac disease panel, and are symptomatic, but get a biopsy and are told they don't have villous atrophy or enough villous atrophy YET, so therefore they don't need to go on a gluten-free diet. This scenario makes my head spin in unattractive ways, as it delays or prevents the only appropriate treatment from occurring. These people are at increased risk for complications such as bowel cancer and lymphoma, osteoporosis, dementia, additional autoimmune diseases and neurological complications that are much harder to treat once the damage is done.

Part 2: Going Gluten Free

Every March, the Columbia University Celiac Disease Center holds a conference, and I attend it every year. It used to be cloaked under the stealthy, ambiguous title of the "Intestinal Immune-Based Inflammatory Disease Symposium," but in 2014 it morphed into the more accurate "Development of Therapies for Celiac Disease" to portray its focus on non-dietary treatment plans for celiac disease.

It was during the 2014 conference that the unthinkable occurred. I was glutened at lunch on the first day. I always looked forward to the food at this particular conference because it had always been safe, delicious, and well presented. My diet had been based on the Paleo principles of meat and fish, fruits and vegetables, and nuts and seeds for the preceding four years, so I choose from the offerings accordingly: meat, salmon, and veggies. But within ten minutes, I knew I had been hit with a gluten stick. My first indicator was the telltale mouth blisters that formed quickly, followed by my stomach roiling. I was in shock. I almost couldn't believe it. I didn't want to believe it. My modus operandi at these conferences is typically to fly under the radar as much as possible until my Tourette's syndrome gets the better of me and I blurt a question in response to something that is so irksome I can't maintain my silence. But in this instance, I was simply stunned.

The next day, one of the executive directors of a national celiac organization and I were talking. She said, "Nadine, I have to ask you a personal question."

"Shoot. Ask me anything," I said.

She responded by telling me she had developed neurological symptoms typical of a gluten exposure. "Did you get symptoms after eating yesterday?" she asked.

I confessed that I had developed mouth blisters almost immediately. By day two of the conference, my urine smelled like an old lady in a nursing home who hadn't had her Depends changed for days. Nice—a urinary tract infection. And a new outbreak of dermatitis herpetiformis across my shoulders and on my back that lasted for several months. In all of my travels and potential hits with gluten at restaurants or friends' houses, or from eating some packaged food, this was by far the very worst exposure to gluten I had experienced since I had been gluten free. Period and hands down.

Most concerning to me was that after follow-up phone calls with the Columbia University Celiac Disease Center registered dietitian in charge of making sure the meals were 100 percent gluten free, she was unable to trace the source of gluten or cross-contamination in the kitchen. Not a confidence builder, to say the least.

Within a week, I was experiencing a new and disconcerting set of symptoms that included having blood in my urine. I ended up having to take antibiotics because that telltale flank pain was getting my attention. Against my best efforts to treat it without antibiotics, I was forced to get a prescription. The autoimmune reaction from the gluten at that day's lunch triggered symptomatic sequelae, a cascade of symptoms that lasted for several months. In the past, if I was accidentally exposed to gluten, I would have symptoms for ten weeks. Two and a half months. I could count the days before my sinuses would clear, my skin would calm down, and my joints wouldn't be achy anymore. This was a new, even lengthier (eight months, to be exact), and very unpleasant experience I hope never ever to repeat ever again. Ever.

As my friend and fellow celiac Paxton says, "People need to understand that the damage to your body happens whether you have symptoms or not. There is no safe amount of gluten we can have." I couldn't have said it better myself.

A gluten-free diet is preventative for so many conditions. As a nurse, it would be unconscionable to not offer a potentially healing diet change to patients who are clearly suffering from "undiagnosable" or "idiopathic" signs and symptoms. Why would anyone want to wait until they had Marsh IV damage, severe intestinal organ damage, or irreversible neurological damage before they were told to go on a gluten-free diet? If we are talking about preventing disease, then adopting a gluten-free diet early is certainly preventative. If you aren't exposed to gluten, you will never develop gluten intolerance, celiac disease, or any of the life-altering or life-threatening complications from untreated celiac disease.

This is a general beginning guide suitable for starting a gluten-free lifestyle. Please keep in mind that everyone is different, and that there are many variables and options. But the critical thing is to remove all wheat, barley, rye, oats, and any derivatives of these grains from your diet *and* your personal care products. Remember that it is not just the "gluten" proteins that can cause problems. You may be sensitized to most, if not all of the various components of wheat and other grains. Plus, the risk of cross-contamination when utilizing any component of gluten grains—such as wheat germ oil in your skincare products—is not worth the potential symptoms or damage (symptomatic or not) that can occur.

Gluten Free All Over: A Special Note

There is a ton of misinformation out there about gluten in skin and personal care products not mattering because unless you are eating the shampoo, lotions, or whatever you happen to be putting on your skin, it just doesn't matter. I beg to differ. This is a topic I am happy to discuss and debate with anyone who disagrees. The status quo from the "experts" is that the gluten protein is too large to get through your skin and into your intestines to cause any damage. One dermatologist even suggested we humans are wrapped in an impervious barrier, like plastic wrap, and therefore, gluten is not a problem. There are several problems with that statement. One is that I am not wrapped in a protective covering of plastic. Two, our skin absorbs everything we put on it directly into the bloodstream, which is one reason we are able to use transdermal medications like nitroglycerin in the emergency department. Nurses have to be very careful not to get it on their skin because it can cause their blood pressure to drop along with the patient's, and it just never looks good when the nurse is lying on the floor while the patient is having chest pain and being worked up for an acute myocardial infarction.

If you're using mascara and—surprise!—your mascara has wheat germ oil in it, you're not just applying that mascara to your eyelashes, but, as we talked about before, directly next to your mucous membrane and potentially your eyeball. Much quicker access to your bloodstream.

Please keep in mind that gluten intolerance and celiac disease are not just damaging to your intestines. An intolerance to the gluten proteins causes not just intestinal, but neurological and skin disturbances and damage. It took me no time at all to figure out that I could change my diet to gluten free all I wanted, but if I didn't also change my personal care products—my shampoo, conditioner, lotions, mascara, lipstick, etc. etc.—then my skin was not going to recover. Once I resolved once again not to listen to the party line, my skin improved rapidly and my DH wasn't raging anymore. If you do not have dermatitis herpetiformis, thank your lucky stars, but do everything you can to potentially prevent an outbreak and further diminish your potential exposure to the grains—even the ones in your personal care products. Trust me, I am a nurse. I give an entire lecture on skin and celiac disease, and it is always well attended.

I now present…

Nurse Nadine's Keys to Going Gluten Free

Start your 100 percent gluten- (all wheat, barley, rye, and oats) and dairy-free diet as quickly as possible.

Here's the deal: I wish someone had told this to me right off the bat. It takes at least six months for your guts to heal, sometimes longer. Going gluten free and dairy free (all mammary milk, goats and sheep included) will speed up the healing process. Start with the goal of being gluten free and dairy free for at least six weeks, and you will see and feel the difference in your health. If you really want to get better as quickly as possible, leap on the Paleo diet and lifestyle. I wish someone had suggested this to me at the get-go. Some people feel better in the first few days, while others don't notice the difference for over a year. Let's say you don't feel better in the early phase, for whatever reason; you are still giving your body the best opportunity to heal.

Most importantly, remember that all it takes is a breadcrumb to trigger an autoimmune response. Once an autoimmune reaction has been triggered, the symptoms can last for days, weeks, or months. If you are still making gluten-containing foods, especially foods that involve using flour, this airborne exposure is more than enough to cause symptoms. This is why cross-contamination is such a huge issue. Some people can tell immediately when they have been exposed to gluten, while some don't get any symptoms. We don't consider this to be to their advantage. The damage occurs whether you are aware of it or not. If you continue to get contaminated with gluten—even a breadcrumb—your intestines will have a difficult time healing.

Take responsibility for your health, but also ask for and accept help.

Changing your lifestyle to accommodate a gluten-free diet can be huge and overwhelming. Those of us at the Gluten Free RN office know. We have been there, made the mistakes, and learned from them. Thinking back, most of us were sick of being sick, tired, grumpy, sleepy... basically, we were the dwarves from Snow White. We needed help, support, and counseling from each other to help us get healthy again.

Take liquid multivitamins every day.

Be certain they are certified gluten free, with no wheatgrass or barley grass. Wheatgrass and barley grass in one liquid multivitamin that was labeled "gluten free" caused one of my lovely clients to have seizures. I currently recommend Country Life multivitamins, but any gluten-free brand will do. In the beginning, consider taking a dose of liquid multivitamins in the morning and at night, always with food, and preferably food with fat in it such as avocados, fish oil, olive oil, eggs or coconut oil.

I recommend liquid vitamins for a number of reasons. They have a higher concentration of vitamins, and they are easier for your damaged intestines to absorb, as they don't need to break down as with a tablet or a capsule. They are necessary for your body to heal and as your body heals, it will need the vitamins available to be absorbed to continue healing. If for some reason you cannot take the liquid form of multivitamins, capsules are the next best option. Try to avoid taking the tablet form of any vitamin or supplement.

Additionally, any other vitamin, mineral, or other supplement you need to take is going to be more easily absorbed in the liquid form.

Consider taking a probiotic if you have EVER taken an antibiotic.

There are many reasons our intestines are unhealthy. Celiac disease tends to be the underlying issue for many of us, but by the time we find out, damage is done that needs to be repaired ASAP. One of the concerns is called small intestinal bacterial overgrowth or SIBO. This can be diagnosed with a breath test for hydrogen and methane. There are several ways to treat SIBO. There is a specific prescription antibiotic, herbal preparations, elimination diets, and probiotics. The probiotics in yogurt or the cheap probiotics at the pharmacy are not enough, however. Visit your local, reputable health food store and get a medium to expensive form of probiotics that typically are required to be refrigerated. I have several brands that I like to use, one being Dr. Ohhira's Probiotics. This is another treatment you can consider doing in the morning and at night at least for the first month or two. And if for some reason you find you are prescribed a course of antibiotics, start taking the probiotic along with the antibiotic, and continue to take the probiotic for at least one to two months after the antibiotic course is done. This is true even for people who don't have celiac disease. Probiotics are also found in fermented foods and beverages such as kombucha, sauerkraut, kimchi and kefir, and they can even help prevent MRSA, *Clostridium difficile*, and other "superbug" infections.

Clean out your kitchen and cupboards.

The best way to start is to determine if your whole house will be gluten free. I highly recommend doing so from the start, for many reasons. It will significantly decrease your risk of cross contamination. You will not feel paranoid in your own home. ("Is there a bread crumb in my mayonnaise jar?") Your family will have the opportunity to support you in your home and they won't have to be constantly concerned about cleaning up the gluten crumbs.

Clean out all the food from your cupboards and give or throw away all the gluten-containing foods (check your spices too), then vacuum and wash the insides of the cupboards. Do this twice if the cupboards contained any gluten flours or pasta. Change all your used wooden cutting boards, rolling pins, and wooden spoons. Either get new wooden ones or replace them with non-porous ones made from granite, stainless steel, or glass. Think about products that don't get scratched and can be cleaned easily and thoroughly. You must change out the toaster. Get a new one that is used only for gluten-free bread. If you have pets, seriously consider feeding them gluten-free or grain-free pet food. This will cut down on the cross-contamination risk, plus your dogs, cats, and other pets will be much healthier.

Wash your hands and produce before you eat.

It is amazing how people can get contaminated from either not washing their hands before they eat or from not washing their fruits and vegetables before they are eaten. If you have any doubts that it matters, just watch what employees eat either in grocery stores before they put out your fresh produce, or even at the farmers market. There are gluten-containing foods everywhere, even around your fresh produce. It is always tempting to eat fresh berries and apples right from the container at the farmers market, but you have to think, *What did the person who picked my produce eat?* (Probably a sandwich!) and, *Did they wash their hands before they touched it?* (Probably not.)

ALWAYS carry snacks.

There is nothing worse than getting stuck without something to eat when you are hungry. Put snacks everywhere: in your purse, in your car, backpack, locker, desk drawers, everywhere. Ideas for snacks are packaged fruit-and-nut bars, bags of nuts, dried fruit, fresh fruit, fruit cups, gluten-free granola, and crackers. If there isn't anything, go without. You will not starve to death in twelve hours. Trust me—you won't.

Avoid cross-contamination as much as possible.

If you share a home with someone who does eat gluten, make a gluten cupboard, or designate a specific area in which to store those products and utensils to avoid cross-contamination as much as possible. Always put gluten-free foods and flours *above* the gluten-containing foods. Designate the upper cupboards as gluten free and the lower cupboards for gluten. If you have the space, designate a completely separate area in the kitchen as gluten free ONLY. Get color-coded utensils, cookware, and dishware that are only to be used for gluten-free cooking and baking. Stainless steel cookware and glass bakeware are easiest to clean. Keep in mind that gluten stays in the air for seventy-two hours and will settle on everything. So if someone makes bread or cookies with wheat flour, that flour is airborne and will cause a dusting in the kitchen.

Remember that eating out is like playing Russian roulette.

Even items without gluten are not safe from cross-contamination if the kitchen still has wheat in it. Most restaurants are not designated gluten free, and very few have designated a gluten-free cooking area. If a restaurant offers gluten-free options, ask lots of questions of the staff, including the chef. It is way too easy to get glutenized, aka "hit with the gluten stick" in a restaurant. Always feel comforted when you see a Gluten Intolerance Group of North America (GIG) or Gluten-Free Restaurant Awareness Program (GFRAP) sign in the window, but still remain vigilant and speak up at all times. Fortunately, I have successfully eaten in restaurants far more times than I can count, but the opportunity of contamination is very real, each and every time. Get comfortable speaking up for yourself regarding your dietary needs. Restaurants are making more of an effort to accommodate people with varied food intolerances and celiac disease, as they should. If there is any question about the food not being gluten free, just don't eat it. It's not worth the risk.

Expect to feel like you can't get enough to eat initially.

Buy and eat the best possible food you can afford and, as long as it's gluten free, eat as much as you want. This is not a joke. Your body has been starved of vital nutrients, possibly for a very long time. It will take some time, effort, and money spent on food to recover, but you will. Eating gluten free is not about calorie counting. Actually, we recommend you eat a good high-fat, whole-foods diet. Eat as much fat as you want. This includes eating bacon and then using the bacon fat to sauté your green leafy vegetables. Because celiac patients don't absorb fat because of the damage that has been done to the intestines, we are typically not able to adequately absorb the fat-soluble vitamins A, D, E, and K.

Pay attention to cravings for food or other items.

This can be a sign of deficiency. If you are craving foods such as avocados, eat as many and as often as you would like. The same goes for any whole food that is good for you. If you are craving sugar, on the other hand, this probably means you are deficient in nutrients (since sugar is not a nutrient, nor is it necessary), and you probably have a yeast or candida overgrowth. If you have a yeast overgrowth, those yeasty beasties are hungry and they want you to eat carbohydrates/sugar to feed them, sneaky little parasites that they are. If you are chewing ice, craving laundry detergent, or eating dirt, you have a pica, which is not good because you are deficient in a nutrient, typically iron or ferrous sulfate, a situation that can cause anemia.

Avoid products manufactured in a facility that also processes wheat.

When I didn't know any better, I did eat products that were manufactured in facilities that also processed wheat. I know better now. Remember what happens to wheat flour when you add water to it? It turns to paste and is very, very difficult to clean from machinery. Plus, as we mentioned, wheat flour remains airborne for up to seventy-two hours, eventually settling on everything in that facility.

Read and ask questions!

Find information from reliable sources, join a support group, and learn as much as you can. Be aware that misinformation is everywhere. If you are confused by the information you have been given, please contact us so that the Gluten Free RN staff can get the correct information to you. We are dedicated to keeping up with current research and information from around the world.

Be careful when you kiss.

Kissing is a common cause of cross-contamination. Either request that your partner/spouse join you in being gluten free or make sure they are brushing their teeth and washing their hands before physical contact. All bodily fluids are potentially contaminated with gluten, especially breast milk. Breastfeeding mothers need to be aware that whatever they are eating is getting transmitted to their baby via the breast milk. If your baby has eczema, colic, failure to thrive, or tummy issues, please look at YOUR diet first.

Be cautious with alcohol and vinegars.

Alcohol and vinegars are a highly contested arena for the gluten-free community. Scientists and doctors have long maintained that all of the gluten proteins have been removed from the alcohol and vinegar in the distillation process. Granted, these products may test gluten free, even to the 10 ppm level; however, many of us that have celebrated this early news with a gin and tonic, whiskey, or any other grain alcohol, have paid the price either with obvious gluten symptoms or with hangovers that are much worse than anticipated. The only two vinegars you need to actively avoid are malt (barley) vinegar and all distilled (with grains) white vinegar. Real apple cider vinegar is slightly more expensive, but well worth the few extra pennies.

Keep in mind that there is never just one celiac in a family.

Once the "primary celiac" has been identified, all first-degree, second-degree, and extended family members need to be notified as soon as possible for initial and follow-up testing. Please contact the Gluten Free RN office for help in determining the best testing for your situation. And please don't rule out spouses and adopted children; get them tested too.

Find a gluten-free buddy to eat and shop with.

Change can be overwhelming, so use the people and resources available to you. There is power in numbers, and a support team is helpful. Studies have shown that people who join a celiac support group adjust to a gluten-free lifestyle more quickly and are able to more easily maintain the changes necessary to regain their health. As more and more people finally get diagnosed, our gluten-free community continues to grow. Find a seasoned gluten-free friend to venture out with to restaurants and the grocery store.

Find a health-care practitioner who can really help you.

Now that you are removing gluten from your diet, the cause of many of your health issues, your body needs supportive care. Find, make appointments with, and hire a supportive provider, including a doctor—either an MD, a doctor of osteopathic medicine (DO), or a naturopathic doctor (ND); look for doctors who practice functional and/or integrative health care—an acupuncturist, a chiropractor, a massage therapist, and so on. You may also find that many of the prescription medications you are taking are no longer necessary, so work with your doctor or health-care provider to continually reassess your medication needs. One of the resources I recommend to find knowledgeable medical practitioners in your area is www.PrimalDocs.com.

Think about keeping a diary and/or food log.

A diary or food log can be a useful tool as you transition into a gluten-free lifestyle. Keeping track of what you are eating and how food makes you feel will help you identify other possible intolerances. Make a list of your current symptoms and how you feel throughout the day. This type of diary will allow you to see progress you have made and help you keep track of your healing process. And remind yourself frequently that this is a process. Your body has been damaged over time, and healing takes time.

Revamp your personal-care lineup.

What do I look for when I am buying gluten-free personal care and skin products? I look for a very clear list of ingredients, and the source of those ingredients. If vitamin E is an ingredient, I need to know where that vitamin E is sourced from, because most vitamin E is sourced from wheat. If I can't tell from the label, I usually will not buy the product. I also look for labeling that states clearly that the product is made with gluten-free ingredients, and that it's been tested to be gluten free. I also make sure I am familiar with the company and the standards they follow to maintain the integrity of their product.

These are some examples of personal care products that I use. No one sends me money to endorse their products. I don't allow any company to give me products to try unless they understand that I am under no obligation to endorse their products, and that if they give me products to try and they cause a problem, I will make that known. These are the products I buy and use without any problems.

- **Desert Essence Organics shampoos, conditioners, lotions and body washes.** The tubes all state in big letters that their product is 100 percent vegan and wheat/gluten free. The shampoos and lotions all smell like fresh fruit, which is pleasant in the morning. None of their products contain any of those other nasty chemicals like parabens or sulfates or petroleum-based ingredients. Plus, just about every grocery store carries this product line, so it's readily available when I am traveling and is not super expensive. When it's on sale, I tend to stock up on my favorite shampoo, Red Raspberry.
- **Red Apple Lipstick.** A fabulous 100 percent gluten-free line of lipsticks, lip glosses, eye shadows, and now mascara. No scary ingredients in any of these products from Houston, Texas. If I am wearing lipstick, it is most likely Red Apple Lipstick. You can find them at many of the gluten-free conferences or order online at www.redapplelipstick.com.
- **Lovely Lady Products.** I fell in love not just with the products but also with the founder of Lovely Lady Products, Cheryl Caspi. She is celiac herself and has risen above every industry standard with her line of personal care products. Cheryl is the stellar, bar-raising entrepreneur of 100 percent gluten-free and everything-else-free products, and she has reached the stratosphere of certifications, awards, and purity for her product line. Cheryl can be found at many gluten-free conferences around the United States. Her products can also be found at many natural grocery stores, and online at www.lovelyladyproducts.com.
- **Primal Pit Paste.** My personal care products underwent a major cleanout and replacement once I realized there was gluten in my bathroom. All except my deodorant, that is. I was trapped into buying potentially harmful deodorants because I had no options other than making

my own. I was saved from a potential DIY deodorant project by Primal Pit Paste. This product is amazing. I normally hate—and I do mean hate—slimy, wet, nasty alternative deodorants that don't work. This product is superior in every way possible. I bought my first stash at the Paleo f(x) Conference in 2014 in Austin, Texas, and I have been successfully converted to a happy and non-stinky Primal Pit Paste user ever since. www.primalpitpaste.com.

- **Primal Life Organics.** This is an amazing product line developed by Trina Felber, RN, BSN, MSN, CRNA. Trina has developed an entire product line of certified organic, Paleo, gluten free, vegan, primal skincare that is purely decadent and fabulous. Trina also offers Primal Pit Sticks in various scents such as lavender (my favorite!), coconut, forest, and several made specifically for sensitive skin. Trina has most recently developed and added an entire cosmetic line to her offerings. To find more information on Trina and her skin care product line, go to www.primallifeorganics.com.

My friend Page also makes what I call my "face crack"—as in I must have a constant and ready supply of my face crack. I don't know how she makes her special secret serums, lotions, and potions that are all gluten free and void of every other nasty chemical I don't want on my skin or near my body, but I am hooked. Her products keep my wrinkles from being so deep set and highly visible. At this point she only makes small batches for friends and family, thankfully one of whom is ME. If she ever decides to offer her products to others, I will definitely be a spokesperson, but for now, I will just thank the Lord Jesus that I have her number on speed dial.

I have what can only be described as "Jack Nicholson-in-*The Shining* eyebrow-raising syndrome." Whatever that muscle group is in my cranium, those muscles are strong. Couple that with post Grave's disease, which caused me to be "bug eyed," or as we say in medicine, suffering from exophthalmos. Once my Grave's disease started to resolve (and yes, that is possible), I started to develop sagging eyelid skin once my eyes began to slowly sink back into my head where they belong. I now have the makings of that particular maniacal look. My eyelid skin literally gets pulled up into several inverted "V" shapes whenever my eyebrows raise in wonderment, skepticism, laughter, or surprise. The fact is, I need plastic surgery to remove the excess skin on my eyelids. I am not even a vain person, nor do I really care. I earned every one of these wrinkles. What I do care about is being able to see through my eyeballs. Also, right now there is no point in buying any eye shadow products because my eyelids are tucked and folded into their own eyelid cave. My mascara will commonly end up on my upper lids, because that's where my eyelids are propped—on my eyelashes! If they are not nipped and tucked into some semblance of a normal position, they will quickly obscure what little vision I have left. I look like a Shar Pei—one of those dogs with an abundance of excess skin. Or a person who has lost an enormous amount of weight. But I haven't. I lost forty pounds, but it wasn't all from my head, thankfully. If anyone is interested, I have considered donating or selling the excess skin from my eyelids to a man who wants to reverse his circumcision. My eyelid skin could be your new foreskin.

Track your progress.

Take a picture of yourself now, in three months, six months, one year, and every year thereafter to track your progress. Wear as few clothes as possible. Take pictures of rashes, bruising, or anything you consider to be a concern. This will help you realize how much healing has occurred. Often, the transformation you can see on the outside is amazing. And you are healing just as much, if not more, on the inside of your body.

You may feel unwell at the beginning as your body detoxifies from gluten and dairy; possible symptoms include headaches, diarrhea, and fatigue. This will clear up, but may reoccur as you heal. You will have very good days, but you may also have miserable ones. Just get through the miserable days and realize the symptoms will pass, and that you will get better. Also, just because you have symptoms similar to your pre-gluten-free days doesn't mean you've been glutened. It could just be that your body is healing, and healing can be uncomfortable at times. Think about a broken bone. It hurts a lot worse the first few days after it's broken, before it starts to heal.

And finally, remember that this is going to take time and energy, so be patient while your body heals.

Stories of Patients (and Patience)

One of my favorite stories is about a very nice, older, big-bellied-with-suspenders-holding-up-his-jeans single farmer man. I gave a class called "Choosing Nutrient Dense Foods When Eating Gluten Free" at a local health foods store. It was an evening class in the rainy winter, and he was the only one who showed up. I have a rule for myself that if even one person shows up, I will proceed with the class. I presented the basic background information on gluten intolerance and celiac disease, then moved on to the core of the information regarding nutrient-dense foods as medicine to heal the body. The farmer listened and asked intelligent questions, and we laughed about his being the only attendee.

Several weeks went by, and he stopped by my office. His suspenders were no longer necessary. His belly was almost flat, and his pants were fitting him much better. "I feel so much better. I lost my belly—it just disappeared!" he laughed. He brought in a few products for me to vet, but otherwise he was fully on board and could not believe the difference. He also recognized that his sister would probably benefit from changing her diet too. He is such a sweet, lovely man, and he's now working on his farm with newfound vim and vigor. More power to him and all who want to feel better, have more energy, and live long and productive lives that allow them to focus on their choice of activities.

Another lovely couple came into my office for a consultation one day, each carrying their own personal baskets of prescription medications: bottles filled with Remicade, Imuran, prednisone, blood pressure medications, and many more. She had been diagnosed with rheumatoid arthritis and he had been diagnosed with Crohn's disease. He had his own business but could not leave the house because he could never be far from a bathroom, ever. He stated he had at least twelve to fifteen bouts of diarrhea a day, so he hired people to do the actual work while he stayed home or in his office, close to the toilet.

The lovely wife explained to me, "I do all of the cooking so he eats what I fix and what I eat."

My recommendation to them was to get both antibody celiac panels and genetic testing for celiac disease. They both were covered by insurance and their doctors agreed to order the tests from Prometheus labs. So they went off, got tested, and came back for an appointment to review the lab results. Her test was gene positive and showed elevated antibodies to gluten. Her doctor had advised her to go gluten free.

He smirked and slid his test over to me on the table. "Here, tell me what this says."

I looked at the test results. "You are not a gene carrier for either the HLA-DQ2 or DQ8 gene and your antibody test is negative. This is a completely negative test for celiac disease," I told him.

He raised his eyebrows, got a glint in his eyes, and said, "Yeah, but I don't have Crohn's anymore! As soon as we got our blood drawn, she started cooking gluten free for both of us. Within a week, I started to get better. Now I only go to the bathroom once or twice a day like a normal person!"

He and his wife cracked up laughing. Both of their doctors were also decreasing the doses of their medications.

"What do you make of that?" he asked.

I responded, "Well, let's just crumple up this paper, toss it into the round file, and stay on a gluten-free diet."

He assured me he would anyway because "she does all of the cooking, so I eat what she makes me."

Now, as I am driving around town, I see him driving his own business' vehicles, and if he sees me first, he honks, waves, and gives me a thumbs-up.

It's important for me to share stories about people who recognize how undiagnosed gluten intolerance and celiac disease has affected their lives. Several of my wonderful clients, friends, and family members have agreed to share their stories because they want to spare other people the pain and suffering they have had to endure, sometimes for years and years. While there are several compelling stories represented here in this book, realize there are hundreds, thousands, and eventually millions of stories that could be told.

Something I started asking people several years ago is to finish the following statement: "I wish I knew I had gluten intolerance or celiac disease..." Each person fills in this statement in their own unique way.

- "...before I had a twenty-pound tumor and ovarian cyst."
- "...before my dad had suffered for over ten years."
- "...so I could have felt this good my whole life."
- "...because I might have whipped Prefontaine in a mile or two or become a Congressman."
- "...before I had multiple miscarriages."
- "...before I had my gallbladder removed."
- "...before I developed insulin-dependent diabetes."
- "...before my migraines took control of my life."
- "...so my kids could have not been exposed to gluten, ever."

Relax. I am not going to try to sell you anything. Not a pill, or a magic cure, or even some gluten-free personal care product. Through my personal story and through the stories of other people, my goal is to convey a sense of hope for your future and the futures of your children and grandchildren. If you recognize symptoms that you suffer with, and if you've been told you're crazy, that you're making your symptoms up, and/or that you have anxiety, depression, chronic fatigue, IBS, fibromyalgia, or any other similarly vague diagnosis, then at least you now have enough information to get started in finding out your own truth. It has taken some of us decades to determine the underlying cause of our myriad, frequently misdiagnosed signs and symptoms. Now you have the benefit of knowing that gluten intolerance or celiac disease are potentially the answer, or at least the missing link, to your health problems.

Analisa's Story (Nadine's Words)

Analisa is my (adopted) daughter Hannah's birth sister. Both of them are stunningly beautiful, brilliant, and socially adept. Several years ago, Analisa and Chris, the kind, handsome, artistically talented brother to Analisa and Hannah, came to Oregon to visit our family for a few weeks in the summer and to spend quality time getting to know their sister. Chris and Analisa asked me what I do as a nurse and I explained my work as the Gluten Free RN. I also explained that Hannah is gene positive and what that potentially means for them. We sat at the kitchen breakfast bar one evening and I essentially presented the "Introduction to Gluten Intolerance and Celiac Disease" class that I have given literally thousands of times. This spurred several questions and multiple conversations.

Shortly after, Analisa came to me and asked me if I knew anything about scalp eczema. Analisa and I went into Hannah's room and Analisa took off her head wrap. I was shocked to see this gorgeous nineteen-year-old's head covered with vitiligo, a depigmentation of her skin tone that was extending onto her forehead, along with deep, crusty lesions and areas where her hair had completely fallen out.

I asked her, "Miss Analisa, what are you putting on your scalp? What hair products are you using?"

Analisa presented me with a large bottle very clearly labeled "WHEAT GERM OIL." I had Analisa place that entire bottle and all of her other personal care products in a big biohazard bag and got it all out of the house. She said that the professional hair people that were doing her hair and selling her those products told her that was just the way her scalp was going to be and that there was nothing to do about it. We quickly replaced all of her hair care and personal care products with gluten-free products and she went on a gluten-free diet, at least for the time she was with us. Within three weeks, her vitiligo, an autoimmune issue, and the lesions were gone, and her hair was starting to grow back in the areas that had previously been essentially bald.

Now, several years since that first visit, Analisa's hair is gorgeous and she keeps it natural, using coconut oil to condition her hair and her skin. She no longer has the stomach issues that had plagued her since before she can remember. We laughed the last time she was in Oregon that she had to come to Oregon and talk to her white mother all those years ago to figure out her African American hair issues. We laughed, but we also realized how not funny her story truly is. There must be millions of people out there who don't know that their scalp and skin issues are related to what they are eating and what they are putting on their skin.

Chris is on a Paleo diet and went with me to Paleo f(x) in Austin last year where he truly shined, and I was extremely proud to introduce him to the Paleo community. He is built like an Adonis after his body composition changed from working out and living a Paleo lifestyle. We are all truly blessed to have each other, and I could not be more boastfully proud of all of my kids.

Katy's Story (Nadine's Words)

I met Katy when I put the word out that I was interested in hiring someone to help me with the office side of RN On Call, Inc. and Gluten Free RN. My businesses were growing, but shockingly, the days were not getting longer to allow me to complete all of the tasks and duties a business owner must accomplish along with taking care of patients, families, supplies, and paperwork. My office had moved from my home to downtown Corvallis on 4th Street, conveniently located under the Darkside… Cinema. My friends from New York still think my location is remarkably appropriate for me.

Katy sat at my desk in a somewhat formal fashion for the initial meet-and-greet to discuss what I was looking for (but that I was not at all optimistic about finding). After conversing with Katy for roughly fifteen minutes, though, I knew I wanted to hire her immediately, which I did, because I am the boss. She told me about herself, her story and why she sought out employment as executive assistant to RN On Call, Inc. & Gluten Free RN. Right off the bat, Katy was a dream come true.

Katy's first day with me was the next day, and it was truly trial by fire. I had to somewhat urgently move one of my clients from the hospital to an assisted-living facility for a temporary stay. Katy brought her truck, boxes, efficiency, and muscles. Not only did I quickly come to love Katy as an employee, I wanted to adopt her.

According to Katy, she was always constipated, dating back to as far as she could remember. She also had abdominal pain so severe that it would cause her to double over and that had sent her to the doctor or emergency department multiple times. Many tests were performed, her blood was drawn, and on paper, Katy looked great. There were many visits to the emergency department when Katy and her family would be told there was nothing wrong with her other than constipation, which those of us in the business refer to as FOS or "full of shit." She would be prescribed enemas and stool softeners, and told to eat a high-fiber diet with lots of grains. Several doctors prescribed pain medication or anti-anxiety medications such as Ativan. This went on for years and years until one trip to the emergency department, which resulted in a surgical consult and a diagnosis of "megacolon." The surgeon deemed Katy's megacolon to be her problem and advised removing it. Katy was nineteen years old at the time. A very real concern was that Katy would end up with a colostomy bag as a nineteen-year-old woman, but thankfully she had an excellent surgeon who was able to remove her colon and successfully anastomose her small intestine or ileum to her rectum. After the procedure, the surgery crew took a picture of Katy's colon in the OR. In the picture, it is being held at each end by a man well over six feet tall. Katy's colon was remarkable and picture worthy because it was three times longer and three times wider than it should have been. A normal colon is approximately three feet long. Katy's colon was well over nine feet long, with a much wider diameter than is ever normal. The doctor also told Katy that all of the nerves in her colon were essentially dead—in hindsight, Katy's megacolon was caused by a neurological disorder, not a lack of fiber in her diet.

With Katy's colon removed, the expectation was that she would get better, but she didn't. As a matter of fact, she started to get worse. She was back in the ED with abdominal pain, diarrhea, and new symptoms. She developed bumps on her legs and was worked up for lupus, sarcoidosis, and other autoimmune diseases. Katy was a full-time student at Oregon State University studying for a nutrition degree, and working at a restaurant as a waitress, and physically, her body was falling apart. On the last day of classes before Katy was due to graduate, Denise Cedar, a registered dietitian from Salem Hospital came and gave a class on celiac disease. Katy said to herself, "Oh my god, that's what I have! I have celiac disease and so does my whole family!" Katy went home, ordered a test online through Enterolab, and lo and behold, her test was positive. No one, not any of the multitudes of doctors that Katy had seen since infancy for her chronic abdominal pain and constipation, had ever tested her for celiac disease. Katy went on a gluten-free diet and started to get better. If she was exposed to gluten through cross-contamination or a missed ingredient, she would vomit and her intestines would shut down. More enemas.

When Katy applied to work in my office, she had recently graduated, and was taking a year off school to work and get healthy before she started her Doctor of Osteopathy program. She was a perfect fit in every way possible as my spunky executive assistant, and she was looking forward to learning and working together in my office. We held classes and meeting, did research, looked for grants, wrote letters to politicians, including the president and Mrs. Obama, made plans for expansion, and investigated developing a certification program for nurses and other health-care professionals. We were very busy.

Katy had a photo of her colon from the OR in which one of the OR staff is holding Katy's colon from end to end—and it is huge. Once I saw that photo, I decided to make Katy's colon famous, so that photo has been shown to thousands of people at my lectures and presentations all over the country. Katy just laughs when I tell her how many people have seen her colon. She wants me to also include a photo of her finishing a marathon or working as a doctor so people can see that she is much improved and healthy. If you haven't seen Katy's famous colon at this point, schedule a class and it will be included in the lecture.

Interestingly, Katy is five feet four inches tall, but her feet are a size ten. Katy should have been over six feet tall. She is a prime example of stunted growth. Because Katy had malnutrition due to her undiagnosed celiac disease, her body couldn't grow. If we can catch children before their bones (epiphyseal plates) seal in adolescence, we can get them to grow to their predetermined height. If not, then stunted growth is damage done that can't be reversed or fixed. I work with many children who are falling off the growth charts or have been diagnosed with a "failure to thrive." One of the first families I worked with years ago came to see me because their child had not grown since she was seven months old, but had just had her first birthday. Her mother was very concerned that her child had not physically grown in five months. She had not grown an inch, gained a pound, popped through a new tooth, or grown out of her shoes or clothes during this entire time.

The mom took the child to pediatricians and was told she, the mother, was too anxious, worrying too much, and perhaps needed to see a counselor. Those pediatricians never really listened to the mom's very real concerns that her daughter was just not growing at all. She was developmentally on track for walking and motor skills but simply not growing. The child was tested for Crohn's disease by one of the practitioners and the test came back positive. The mom was frantic because the diagnosis of Crohn's disease in a one-year-old is essentially a death sentence. I contacted the practitioner who ordered the Crohn's test, explained that there is significant genetic overlap between Crohn's and celiac disease, and would she please test the child for celiac, both with an autoimmune panel and the genetic testing? She agreed to order the additional tests.

Once the blood was drawn and the cheek swab obtained, the mom put the child and all of her other children immediately on a gluten-free diet. She also made an appointment with a pediatric gastroenterologist in Portland, Oregon. That appointment was scheduled seven weeks in the future. When the appointment day arrived, the mom took the child to the appointment with the lab results. The pediatric gastroenterologist took note of the results, which were positive for celiac disease, and started the physical exam. After simply changing the child's diet to gluten-free food, she had grown five inches, popped through four new teeth, increased her shoe size, and no longer suffered with "belly aches" all of the time. The mom had previously been told by multiple pediatricians that 30 percent of children just have belly aches, but that we don't know why and she would simply grow out of them. Whoa.

The pediatric gastroenterologist examined the child and told the mom, "She has celiac disease. I am not going to do an endoscopy. She has celiac disease, and so does your whole family. Just stay gluten free."

Simple, yet it took months of pain, agony, suffering, and torture to find out that this sweet little pixie of a child was not capable of growing because her intestines were damaged from the gluten-containing food in her diet.

Does this story sound familiar to you? Do you know children who are short in stature, are not growing or developing, are slow to respond, are irritable or angry, are picky eaters, are unable to focus on their school work, have rashes, are unable to sleep, are wetting their bed, suffering from delayed puberty, osteoporosis, strokes, arthritis, or muscle pain, have eating disorders, or only eat carbohydrates or "white foods"? Please be an advocate for these children and find a practitioner who will appropriately test them for gluten intolerance and celiac disease

One of Katy's and my proudest accomplishments occurred during her tenure at Gluten Free RN. We held two meetings at the public library in Corvallis. Our intent was to match up investors with people who wanted to start a gluten-free restaurant. We wanted a totally 100 percent gluten-free restaurant to open up in town so that we could go eat there. I had no delusions about doing that myself. I very well may be ambitious, but I am not inclined to challenge myself to open up a restaurant. I was not made to own and/or operate a restaurant. I know I very much appreciate going to restaurants and have nothing but gratitude for restaurant owners who make a point of feeding me safely, but I have no delusions about owning or running one.

So we held these meetings, and people came and voiced their opinions of what they wanted in a gluten-free restaurant. Katy's dad, Sandy McHenry, came to be supportive and to take notes on the whiteboard for us. Sandy, though, has a long history as a barbecue master and catering barbecue events for large groups, and it did not take long before we both could see the hamsters spinning in his brain.

Both of Katy's parents, Sandy and Lynda, are some of the most gracious and welcoming people I have ever met. I was invited on multiple occasions to have dinner with the McHenry family and whoever the other guests of the evening were. Lynda and Sandy are adept at networking, supporting a community, and interconnecting groups of people that need to meet but just don't know it yet. Lynda is a genius at making connections. The idea of family/group dinners and feeding people was not a new concept to either of them.

Sandy's first idea was to open a gluten-free grainery to provide millet, teff, quinoa, and other gluten-free grains. He decided he needed a test kitchen. Out of that first attempt came the first Eats & Treats Café, a tiny restaurant with an impossibly small kitchen, off a busy highway, but turnkey with all of the necessary equipment ready to go. Several weeks were spent on a thorough cleaning, stocking, recipe development, and revamping the space so that the café could open for business. When the café did open, it was to resounding support from the gluten-free communities near and far. The food was amazing and totally gluten free. Kids would come into the café for the first time and their parents would tell them they could have anything in the restaurant they wanted, anything. These are kids who have been told repeatedly what they can't have, and here is a place where everything is safe.

These kids would press their noses to the bakery case and just cry. "Really? Anything I want?"

"Yes, everything in the case is safe for you to eat!"

Shortly after Sandy and Lynda opened their gluten-free restaurant, they expanded and doubled the space. Within a year, they closed the first restaurant and moved a few miles down the highway to Philomath, Oregon, remodeled a space four times larger than the first restaurant, and have been a raging success ever since. They have an extensive menu that highlights Sandy's barbecue prowess and offers many bakery options, and the restaurant always provides gracious and fun company. I can easily eat Paleo there, and others are perfectly happy regardless of their particular food intolerances or preferences.

After a very productive, fun, and educational year, Katy went away for medical school, but she returns frequently to see her family, and me, of course.

Katy's Story (Katy's Words)

> As far back as I can remember, I had stomachaches. My mother always gave me castor oil, which seemed to help, and none of us thought much of it.
>
> "Possible appendicitis," the doctor said, standing over my acute abdomen. "We'll need a CT." After I was scanned, my parents and I sat in a room with the doctor as he went over the images with us. They turned up something none of us expected: I had an enlarged colon. The cause of my acute pain, which had since subsided, was being labeled as a "resolved volvulus." The size of my colon had allowed it to twist and untwist on its own. I was sent home and didn't think much more of it until two years later.
>
> I traveled to Europe for the first time on my own following high school graduation. The thrill of being alone was only magnified by the deliciousness of all the food with which I was presented. In my later years at home, my mother had adhered to the ever-popular low-carb diets; bread, pastas, and cereals were just something we did not eat a lot of. And now here I was, surrounded by more pasta, pizza, and beer than I could imagine. It was after two weeks of this that I began to feel ill. I became sluggish at first, writing it off as the summer heat, followed by downright ill. My stomach gnawed all the time, cramping, aching, from the time I woke up to the time I went to sleep. I stood hunched over, became restless while sitting, anything I could do to relieve the pressure. Finally, after a kind Greek pharmacist took pity on me, I took a box of laxatives and felt some relief. Still painful, still tender, still sluggish, but improved.
>
> Returning home, I started college. Yep: more pizza, more pasta, more beer. The pain never left, and I found that the only way to poop was to take some extra-strength colon cleansers; most

over-the-counter laxatives didn't touch me. None of it, however, stopped the stomachaches. They kept on gnawing. My friends used to joke that they couldn't get me excited or it would start up again. And then there was the weight loss. Despite my audacious college diet, my normal-sized 5'4" frame had dropped an extra 15 pounds. I tried giving blood, but was always turned away for anemia. My hair started falling out. My periods stopped. My days consisted of class and coming home to lie on the floor of my dorm room, curled up. All of my energy was zapped. I became an 18-year-old with less stamina than my 80-year-old grandmother. And then the doctor visits started.

First, I saw a nurse practitioner, who looked at my diet history and decided to give me a trial of Prilosec, for treatment of reflux. No relief. My mother gently reminded me of my previous volvulus attack, which she thought might be related, and so I took it up with another physician at student services. They did an abdominal X-ray, and the doctor actually jumped back when he saw the results—that colon was huge! No wonder my stomach always hurt, and was always distended.

Over Thanksgiving, I met with a gastroenterologist who took one look at my images, touched my stomach, and told me not to worry but to spend more time drinking and smoking like the other kids my age. Another consultant was so worried of the risk of volvulus that she advised me not to return to college, not to travel in the future, and to avoid any risky activities or overexertion.

Back to college I went with no answers, and back to the student services doc, who made a final decision: surgical consult. The surgeon tested me for nearly everything: several colonoscopies, CTs, pills of white rings that could be tracked on x-ray, x-rays while I was using the toilet, gastroenterology visits, psych visits. At the end of the day, they all came to one conclusion: my colon did not work. Whether it stopped working first and became enlarged second or vice versa was unknown. But it would never work, and it had to come out.

I ended the first year of college and went into surgery. The surgery tech took a picture while holding up the longest colon he had ever seen. One week of rehab in the hospital, followed by about two months to get back to my baseline after my recovery was blunted by a smoldering abscess. And I began to feel better.

My stomachaches had largely stopped, and I was no longer bed bound in the evenings, though I wouldn't consider myself overly active either. About six months later, the stomach pain returned, aggressively. Back into the hospital I went for a colonoscopy and a repeat CT, all showing nothing. Return of the "resolving volvulus," it was called. Except that this began to happen every six months, with intermittent abdominal pain in between.

Beginning of senior year. I had switched my major to nutrition, taken all of my medical school prep classes, served as president of a few public health clubs, done research in reproductive sciences, and published a thesis. Yet all the while, I never felt great. At baseline, I was better following my surgery, without the severe, "popping at the seams" pain, but still persistently aching. Still persistently tired.

Halfway through fall semester, I had a kidney infection. I received adequate treatment and two days later boarded a plane, erythromycin in hand, for a conference in Philadelphia. On the second day, I noticed some lumps on my legs. They felt warm and tender to the touch and were darkened and raised. I couldn't remember hitting my shins on anything, and I wasn't a big bruiser, so I thought them odd. Over the next couple of weeks, the lumps grew in number and size, covering my shins. I developed aching joints in my knees and ankles, leaving me with a limp. And my lower back hurt so badly in the mornings, it took a good fifteen minutes to pull myself out of bed. I also had a lurking low-grade fever. Back to student health services, where the doctors were beginning to be more than familiar with me. I thought it odd they chose to do a chest X-ray, until the doctor looked at the results and uttered an "a-ha": Löfgren's syndrome, a rare autoimmune disease, not usually seen in young females. I opted to not treat, and within a few months the mysterious illness left... But the stomachaches stayed.

During my last class of senior year, a guest speaker came in to talk about a disorder called "celiac disease." As she talked about this diarrhea-predominant disorder, I started considering it for my brother. He'd had IBS-like symptoms all of his life, but maybe there was another cause? I went home and started to do more research on my own so I could call him to get tested, but the more I read, the more I realized that he wasn't the only one fitting the symptom list: gastrointestinal issues, fatigue, amenorrhea, anemia, autoimmune disorders. Back one last time to student

> health services, where the nurse practitioner referred me to an online lab to get tested.
>
> Two weeks later, when my results came back, I called my confused parents, crying and exuberant at finally knowing what was wrong with me. One month later, all the gluten had been kicked out of my diet. One year later, I ran my first marathon and started medical school.

Katy's Recent History (Nadine's Words)

Katy has been in her first-year internship as a primary care physician and is very excited to be seeing patients. Just a short while ago, I began getting frantic phone calls from Katy's parents. Katy had been eating food from the hospital and, unbeknownst to Katy, they were putting the bacon on bread to soak up the bacon fat. So the bacon was completely unsafe for Katy or any other unsuspecting celiac. Katy was probably getting other cross-contamination with gluten, but she was too busy being a stellar family practice doctor and taking care of everyone else but herself. Katy went to see a doctor because she had been experiencing excruciating abdominal pain along with "constipation," which Katy knows is not good a good sign. She presented to be seen, was sent to radiology for an x-ray of her abdomen, and was told she had a megacolon.

She responded, "That's really interesting, because I no longer have a colon; it was removed."

"Oh."

After several angst-filled days of inpatient hospitalization, Katy's intestines didn't explode and eventually cleared. Thankfully, no surgery was performed. Katy's records all very clearly declared her celiac status, and Katy herself and her vigilant family and friends were very vocal about having no gluten in her room or anywhere near Katy. In order to be discharged, though, Katy had to eat something before she could leave. What did the hospital staff bring on a tray for Katy to eat before she could be discharged? Cream of Wheat.

Kim's Story (Kim's Words)

When I began my employment at the Gluten Free RN in January 2011, I knew nothing about celiac disease—or gluten, for that matter. The initial part of my interview for the position was sitting in on Nadine's "Introduction to Celiac Disease and Gluten Intolerance" class. Wow. I was amazed and intrigued by what I heard and learned in that hour of time! I was especially intrigued because of the digestive challenges my family has faced on my dad's side of the family…

I am one of six from my dad's family to have an ileoanal anastomosis surgery—a very invasive surgery that basically removes the entire large intestine and then creates an internal "J-pouch" with the lower part of the small intestine. We have always been told we have a rare, inherited condition called familial adenomatous polyposis (FAP), yet the true cause of this condition has never been fully understood or explained to me by medical professionals. This condition can cause hundreds or even thousands of polyps to grow in the colon and rectum, usually starting by your mid-to-late teens. The polyps potentially have a high probability to develop into colon cancer or rectal cancer, so the surgery is seen as a means to prevent this. My fraternal grandfather, who did not have this surgery, died around age forty-nine of colon cancer. I never even had the chance to meet him.

In Nadine's class, I learned that celiac disease is also genetic, chronic, autoimmune, and digestive. And, guess what? It (usually) impacts the lining of the digestive tract, greatly compromising the villi that line the small intestine. When these are compromised, it can lead to "leaky gut," which limits nutrient absorption and can also cause the intestinal walls to "leak," allowing toxins, unhealthy microbes, and even partially digested food into the bloodstream. Hello, inflammatory/autoimmune symptoms and/or diseases. (FAP???) The similarities between what I was now learning about celiac disease/gluten intolerance and what I had been told for years about FAP were uncanny, and I was ready to learn more!

By the end of February 2011, after hearing miraculous story after story, I made the decision to go both gluten and dairy free in one fell swoop. Initially, I had some terrified thoughts of, "What will I eat?!", but in no time I had swapped out my snacks and meal staples for "safe" foods and was on my way. Almost immediately, my energy, stamina, thinking, memory, and digestion improved. The past days of needing a nap by noon were long gone, and I was better able to mentally manage my schedule and life. My lab results were also improving and, as a side benefit, I was becoming leaner and more fit.

I had also begun to switch out some snacks for my husband and kids at home for gluten-free options. But by about six months into my new eating plan, I began to feel guilty that I was eating this way but my family was not. I decided and then announced to my family that we all would go gluten free for one month… to "give it a try" (yeah, not the truth, but I was trying to be sneaky)! My kids, in particular were *not* happy about this… but, I'm Mom, and so that's what we were doing. I found yummy gluten-free alternative recipes or modified regular ones with gluten-free ingredients—like homemade gluten-free chicken nuggets, gluten-free mac and cheese, and gluten-free brownies, which now are preferred to "regular" brownies!

Despite the initial struggle with my kiddos, we maintained the gluten-free diet for a month… and for a couple more weeks, when suddenly my son declared, "Wait! It's been more than a month!"

I casually said, "Oh, it has?" (I knew it had, but I was still in sneaky mode.) "Well, I think we're just going to keep eating this way."

It's not nice to say this but, prior to our diet change, sitting down to do homework with my son was a very unpleasant experience in which my husband and I expended *way* more time and energy on the task than our son did. But guess what? Our son now basically manages his own study time—even utilizing any free time at school to do work!!! Yes, we still help him when he requests it, but he really has taken over the reins on his school work, *and* has been on then honor roll since then, *and* has glowing comments from his teachers on his work ethic, attitude, and use of in-class time!

Additionally, our daughter had been experiencing major fatigue, exhaustion, and mood swings, was catching colds frequently, and even had some warts on her foot that, despite several attempts by a doctor to freeze them, wouldn't resolve. She had been on a gluten-free diet for some time already, but due to these issues, her doctor suggested she go on an elimination diet for several weeks. During this period, along with gluten, she also avoided sugar, eggs, dairy, and corn. At the end of the time period, she had labs redrawn (which showed improvement), the warts disappeared (and have not returned since!), she's enjoyed a much stronger immune system and far fewer colds, and her moods are more stable.

As for me, I have also evolved in my eating plan. I now eat a Paleo (nuts, seeds, meats, fruits, and veggies) diet about ninety percent of the time and allow for occasional gluten-/dairy-free snacks or goodies. I switched to this diet about six months after I initially went gluten-/dairy-free and I noticed even more improvement in my energy and brain clarity, and even saw a significant shift in my body composition; I lost some more weight and have become leaner yet stronger, without adding more exercise or training to my regimen. I have learned that, like life, this is a process... not a destination. What works well today, works well today—but next month, year, etc., might require tweaking based on where my body is at in the healing process at that point. I am so thankful for the improved health and well-being we are enjoying due to our diet change. My hope is that you and many others will experience it as well!

Kim's Story (Nadine's Words)

Between Katy and Kim having had their bowels removed and resected, I decided to make that one of the job requirements to work in the Gluten Free RN office. When we post a job opening on Craig's List next time, it will say, "Must have had part of your small intestine or colon removed in order to be employed by Gluten Free RN." I am certain that is in no way is discriminatory, and I am employing people who are missing body parts and organs. Where else are they going to work?

Amy's Story (Amy's Words)

I think my story is important to tell because it's not the typical one. My children and I don't have strong gastrointestinal reactions to eating gluten. We never tested positive to celiac disease. If we do get "glutened," we can't tell right away, and our reactions are minimal. So for the longest time, I thought we all just had a sensitivity to gluten. The more I learned, the more I realized we could have celiac disease. We could be those people who fly under the radar, whose symptoms are in the middle of the range and who most doctors would never think have celiac disease. This is a problem because until my husband and I tested positive for the gene, until I started to put the pieces together of my health puzzle (which really are not complex), I was not serious about being gluten free. I now know better.

This is how it started. My daughter was just over twelve months old. She was developing some eczema on her thighs. Her pediatrician said "keep an eye on that." I will never forget it because it was the beginning of this journey, more or less. The signs were always there but I didn't know what they meant. Without getting too personal, all of the signs were in the bathroom. Being regular is such a simple indicator of your health (even if you think you are healthy). Back to my daughter. Her eczema just kept getting worse and worse. We tried over-the-counter creams. They didn't work. She was tested for allergies. None. She was prescribed steroid creams (yes, for a baby), which worked only very temporarily. Then, one person said one thing to me: "Maybe it's a food intolerance."

That led me to getting her tested, which led to a diagnosis of leaky gut; which led me to looking at test results, which led me to try to figure out how to feed a twenty-month old foods free of gluten, dairy, eggs, and about ten more things. Ay yai yai! Well, that has led me to today. We are a gluten-free, mostly dairy-free and soy-free, and almost Paleo household. But, it's taken eight years of ups and downs, learning, trying new things, and in the end, being persistent.

The first year of a gluten-/dairy-/egg-free diet was challenging. I was motivated to try new recipes, make changes, talk to people, and learn as much as I could. I did the best I could with the resources I had. I started teaching cooking classes at this time and incorporated gluten-free foods into the repertoire. A year into teaching, I tried gluten free for myself, only because I wanted to understand what people had to deal with. Does this sound familiar? There's nothing wrong with me! I'm fine. I don't have a problem with gluten.

After four days of being gluten free, I realized I no longer had my normal tummy aches I had before I went to the bathroom. Then, about two months later, I noticed I wasn't so tired every day at 3 p.m.; I stopped having that second cup of coffee. Then I realized I was sleeping better (related to not being so tired). It went on and on with little changes. My skin looked better. I lost weight (mostly because I changed what I was eating). And when I did eat gluten, my reactions were becoming worse. I didn't like it one bit.

A year later, my son complained of tummy aches here and there. He was tested for celiac disease, which came back negative, but another test showed he was sensitive to gluten. I took him off of gluten and two weeks later, all of his symptoms went away. I looked at my daughter, whose skin was still irritated. At the time we were trying fish oil, which was not fully effective. She went back on a gluten-free diet. My husband didn't have much choice but honestly, he feels better too.

In early 2014, my husband and I tested positive for the genetic test. That's when we got serious, and that's when my daughter's skin finally cleared up. This was seven years after we started.

In addition, after more testing, we realized my daughter does much better being dairy free as well. We keep her egg consumption to a minimum. Soy bothers me almost as much as gluten, so I avoid it. Since going off of dairy two years ago, I no longer have mucus in my throat or nose and no longer get sinus infections.

My children do not miss school. I mean ever. The last time I kept them home, it was for a slightly runny nose. I gave them a rest day. I have to think this is all connected.

I'm doing the best I can and treat them as if they have celiac disease, but I'm not perfect. There are things I miss. But it's okay, because they are happy, healthy kids. I learn from mistakes, fix them, and move on. So if someone says something to you, or you read this book and you decide to give it a try, stick with it and don't give up. Good luck on your journey.

Deb's Story (Deb's Words)

What I endured: It was right before Thanksgiving, in November 2007. I had been covered in a painful, blistering, burning, fiercely itchy rash for months, and I just felt sick, again… I tried to figure out what was wrong… research… doctors… health professionals… I knew it was something I was doing to myself, but no answers came…

This rash covered my entire back, chest, and arms, including my wrists, and behind my knees. My skin looked like it had been burned. Nothing helped. My nurse practitioner told me to use Benadryl.

I asked another nurse friend to take a look. She asked me some questions and took a brief look, then said, "Looks like dermatitis herpetiformis. You should get tested for celiac disease, then seriously consider a gluten-free diet for a month and I can help you."

So I started my gluten-free journey towards getting my good health back, admittedly with some challenges. The good news is most symptoms disappeared quickly and are gone! From my own experience, our medical professionals wait way too long to test for gluten sensitivity and celiac disease. I have medical records in *dozens* of medical offices across this country documenting symptoms like GERD, stomach pain, brain fog, burping, farting, indigestion, hair loss, skin rashes and dryness, eczema, heartburn, chronic aches and pain, muscle pain and swelling, mouth sores, yeast overgrowth, cold sores, chronic influenza-like pain, fibromyalgia, fatigue, memory loss, life-long insomnia, depression, anxiety, lactose intolerance, pelvic pain, thyroid disease, constant hunger, and more. Often, one issue would resolve while another mysteriously appeared or reappeared. It was pure TORTURE!

For at least two years, I had such severe brain fog, I couldn't read or write; numbers were indecipherable codes. I could barely take care of myself, let alone raise two children and manage a household. Not one doctor ever tested me for gluten sensitivity or celiac. In fact, my intelligence and requests for answers were dismissed and meds were prescribed, some of which I refused to take. That's another story…

I want you to know that I have always been my own health

advocate and am well read in nutrition, doing my very best to be and stay healthy. My health was so poor that I could have been on disability. I refused that life, and knew the clues for good health were there. I would figure it out. I had counted on the medical doctors to help me find a cause to my health issues (thus the hefty stack of medical records). Do you know that doctors are not generally taught the connection between foods and health? They are not trained in nutrition??

What I learned was that I had the answer all along. I learned to trust my gut and crack the code by listening to my body and figuring out some things myself and to look for support in the right places. I believe that early diagnosis of gluten intolerance would PREVENT many diseases. I feel that testing needs to be done at birth and if not, at annual exams. So, get tested, and test your family. If there is even a clue that gluten may be an issue, stop eating it. Be done with it. You now have information that I wish I had as a young adult, and that I wish my parents had when I was a child. No excuses. Take responsibility. Live a longer and healthier life with your children and your families.

In the beginning, I still remember how overwhelmed I was once I fully realized what going gluten free meant. It was not easy back then, and information on what the diet entailed was hard to find, but my very life depended on it. I cried at grocery stores, not knowing what foods were safe and which ones had poisonous gluten in them. Wheat is everywhere, and in and on foods you would not believe! I relied heavily on Nadine's advice and resources.

My thyroid and ovaries never did recover from the damage eating gluten caused. But otherwise, I have healed extremely well and am the healthiest I have EVER been! Today, I focus on preparing and eating whole foods, not processed foods. I feel better and am much healthier, avoiding grains, dairy, sugars, legumes, and processed foods, and always avoiding gluten! I am eating mostly Paleo. So, yes, it can be done! My life depends on it, and maybe so does your children's, your own, or those of other family and friends. If you are in denial, knock it off. Get the facts. Share this information with people you know who have health complaints, no matter how small. Gluten can kill, cause degenerative, debilitating disease and cancers, and a miserable life. Those of us who have been on this journey can help.

Doug's Story (Nadine's Words)

Doug has been in my life as a dad of one of my daughter's friends through elementary school. Doug, a physician's assistant, very handsome, and his lovely wife, Joanne (now a registered nurse), were great about dropping their daughter off at our house or gathering the kids for a play date. Despite the fact that Doug and I were both in the medical community, we didn't cross paths all that often if it didn't involve our kids. Shortly after my diagnosis, our girls were scheduled to go away to fifth grade camp before they graduated into middle school which included us as parent chaperones. The group all went to camp on the Northern Oregon coast on buses, but I had to complete a twelve-hour day shift and decide if I was going to make the three-hour trip that night or sleep in my own bed and make the trip in the morning. I opted to sleep in my own bed, get up ridiculously early, and arrive before breakfast.

I was petrified about trying to eat gluten free at camp. This was going to be my first trip outside of my house or other environments in which I felt comfortable controlling my access to safe food. I panicked, and brought along four bags of gluten-free groceries, supplies, and my own pans, all for two nights. Good thing I drove myself, because my supplies barely fit along with everything else I was instructed to bring. I was still shell-shocked, learning and relying on dubious things I was reading on the Internet.

I will admit it now, but I actually had a "breakdown" in which I felt the overwhelming sadness of not fitting in, anxiety, and *Why? Poor me*! I had to excuse myself and go cry into my pillow on a bunk bed while hunkered in my sleeping bag in a thankfully empty cabin. I felt like a fifth grader instead of a parent! I sobbed and snorted and sobbed some more before I pulled myself together enough to rejoin the group before dinner. To my utter amazement, one of the volunteers turned out to be a chef who knew how to cook gluten free, and he totally made me my own stunning pans of gluten-free food! I was flabbergasted and overwhelmed with gratitude. I quizzed him on cross-contamination and the few other buzzwords I knew to ask, and he schooled me on how to communicate clearly and assured me he would make my camping trip tasty and safe for me. Sweetest man ever. I could now join the rest of the kids in activities and adventures and did not have to feel sorry for myself anymore.

One of my assigned activities was on the dock helping kids to fish, and the other parent assigned with me was Doug. Even though I was still in the early stages of learning, I had already given a few classes in my community on celiac disease, so despite my trepidation, I was spreading my wings as a teacher with a new specialty. Doug asked me questions about what I was learning, and he related some of his own symptoms that had been concerning him for a long time, including a rash on his hands, elbows, and knees, as well as asthma. I was in the early stages of encouraging everyone to get tested, and my fervor was kindled by the symptoms that Doug had recounted. I made suggestions for testing and gave him as much information as I had at that time. I was encouraged and felt a wee bit more confident after I spoke with Doug. Forging a previously untested path in the medical community is fraught with potential pitfalls, but Doug seemed to at least listen and be interested.

Frequently, at this point, most of my friends in the industry of medicine, or even those outside the medical field, were rolling their eyes or practicing avoidance behavior when they saw me coming. They avoided me as if I was going to try to sell them Amway. But I was undeterred. I was on a mission. Certainly, if this had happened to me, it was happening to other people. I had been very nearly missed despite my laundry list of typical and atypical signs and symptoms for years. My years of triage, recognizing sick people and acting accordingly were kicking in, full gear.

After elementary school, our girls went to different middle schools and high schools, but we would run into each other at events or parties. Doug and Joanne would tell me that the gluten-free diet had helped Doug with his rash, but he never really got tested and was back to eating gluten, though less than he had been eating before.

Several years went by without any significant communication. Joanne then posted on Facebook that Doug was in the hospital and was pretty sick, and that he would need to talk to ME very soon. What follows is Doug's recount of his life-changing event that led him to my office and essentially a Paleo lifestyle. When I get people who are critically ill, just out of ICU or the hospital, I now cut to the chase and put them immediately on a version of the Paleo diet, if they agree. They get better faster and more completely, with less suffering. I truly wish someone had suggested a Paleo diet to me when I was first diagnosed in 2006.

Doug's Story (Doug's Words)

> Early morning, January 21, 2014. Before I took Spencer to school, I had my first bloody bowel movement ever. A little shocking. At the time, I was not experiencing any other symptoms. Later that morning while at work, I had two more episodes of bloody diarrhea. I went home early. The blood continued to be expelled about every two hours, and there was a point where it stopped for a while. I was eating fine and still had no other symptoms. I went to bed thinking it would be over in the morning.
>
> Six a.m., January 22, 2014 saw the continuation of the bleeding. Still no pain or significant cramping. Finally told Joanne and she immediately got on the phone to "her people" at work. Several hours later, after chugging a liter of bowel prep, the double scope ensued. I had no discomfort and the news was a mix. Nothing significant on EGD [esophagogastroduodenoscopy] (although they said I had what looked like EE [eosinophilic esophagitis]) and my colon was pristine. Where was the blood coming from? Everyone was perplexed. Still having bloody diarrhea, I was admitted to the hospital. They gave me fluids and checked labs again. Blood count falling. I had a Tech99 scan to look for the source of the bleeding. Nothing! I went back to my room and waited. Joanne and the kids came and kept me company for several hours. Labs again. And again, my H&H (hematocrit and hemoglobin) going down. I remained NPO [Nil per os or nothing by mouth] since the colonoscopy/EGD and still no pain but a swooshing sensation began in my head. My last bloody bowel movement was at about 8:30 p.m. on the twenty-second.
>
> The next morning I was discharged, thinking the bleeding had stopped and my blood count had stabilized. A little weak but not

bad, I went to the GI office to swallow a pill camera to try and see if we could catch a glimpse of what might be gong on. At noon, the camera went down and I was fitted with gear to pick up the signal coming from the camera and capture the pictures. Still no symptoms, but hungry at this point. Had some soup and about six hours later, the blood once again came. Back to the hospital we go.

This time I was starting to feel a little dizzy and a slight headache began. More labs and tests. Another Tech99 scan. This time the bleed was visualized. The pictures from the pill camera were downloaded and the bleed was visible. Along with a stricture, ulcers, and a patency capsule I swallowed yesterday. Don came in and gave me the news. Surgery. A laparoscopic partial small bowel resection was done about 2 p.m. on Friday January 24. No complications.

A few hours later, the news started pouring in. "Looks like Crohn's," Don said.

At this point, my blood count was quite low and I could really tell. Dizziness, the swooshing, and a headache! Got blood and felt better and began clear liquids the next day. Two days post-op, I felt better and wanted the hell out of the hospital. Still dizzy but advancing diet on schedule. Monday, January 27 was tolerable. Was eating solids and drinking TONS of water as to not get dehydrated. I was also peeing at an unprecedented rate. Seemed like I could keep up, but thought with the amount of water I was consuming, who could get dehydrated! Tuesday about three a.m., I awoke to severe dizziness and the pounding headache. Took a shower at six a.m. thinking the bleeding may have started again since I was so symptomatic. Almost passed out twice and Joanne stuck her head in and said, "What the hell are you doing?"

Something was not right, and I needed to go the ED. Off we went. Labs and IV fluids. Dilaudid was given for pain control. Labs looked okay and the liter of fluid made me feel better. Did well after that.

Since high school, I'd had asthma and bad skin. Dry spots on elbows and knees as well growing up. I started taking Advair once a day approximately a dozen years ago and really had no problems. Many puffs of the albuterol inhaler over the years, but very sporadic. One trip to urgent care for a breathing treatment several years ago. I think I had a mild case of bronchitis as well. In addition to the asthma, I had itchy ears! Itching and dry, scaly skin in the ear canals and intermittent scaly patches behind my right ear and on the right side of the bridge of my nose. Lots of hydrocortisone and other creams only did so much, and the flares were unpredictable. I tried, on several occasions, to only take the Advair every other day. No no. Wheezing ensued. Back to every day. But just once a day. I also battled reflux for as long as I remember, and was actually able to cut down on the PPIs [proton pump inhibitors] to just a few times per month in the past year due to losing a little weight, exercising more regularly, and watching the diet. I felt the PPIs were not good for me and stopped taking them altogether about two months ago. If I had reflux, I would drink a few ounces of water with baking soda dissolved in it. Boom! Worked great. I didn't have to do that all that much—perhaps a few times monthly.

Fast-forward to after the small bowel surgery and the Crohn's diagnosis. I was doing research on Crohn's while still in the hospital and came across a web site for something called the specific carbohydrate diet (SCD). Interesting indeed. The lady who began this many decades ago said she cured her young child of inflammatory bowel disease (IBD) on this diet. I was determined not to take the toxic and dangerous drugs doctors are now prescribing for Crohn's, so I thought I would give it a try until I could do further research.

Follow-up with the GI doc was interesting. The diagnosis was discussed, as were the recommended treatment options. From his point of view, Crohn's disease needed to be treated aggressively and for one's lifetime. This meant two different drugs with side-effects that would make your head spin. In addition, the substantial cost of said drugs was equally as dizzying. As the visit went on, I was adamant about not taking the drugs and asked many questions. The most significant question I had was how was the success or failure of the drugs to be monitored? I explained to the doc that before I started bleeding, my GI complaints were far and few between. I had belly discomfort on maybe a half dozen occasions over as many years. On these occasions, I had severe, sharp abdominal pain with mild nausea and twice vomited. I recall one trip to the ED in 2007. I had severe abdominal pain, nausea, and vomiting over and over. I was sent for a CT, which showed a partial small bowel obstruction (SBO) but nothing more, and a surgical consult was not indicated. I recovered and followed up with a general surgeon. No definite reason for the SBO was found and I went on my way. I had more, what I am calling partial SBO, episodes as stated previously, but nothing as significant as in 2007. I finally wised up to the feelings I had prior to these episodes and simply stopped eating or drinking anything for many hours and recovered without incident. The main topic of drug surveillance was uninteresting to the GI doc, and when I asked about dietary changes he basically laughed.

He said, "You could have the strictest diet in the world and it would perhaps have a two percent benefit of helping inflammatory bowel disease." He went on to "sell" the drugs and how well they worked for many people.

I asked another question. "How many people choose dietary changes over drugs when facing a Crohn's diagnosis?"

He said none.

I knew what I had to do, and it was not take the drugs.

The specific carbohydrate diet (SCD) was challenging on many levels. The education on which foods I could eat and the ones to avoid took time. I felt like I was always going to the market for fresh produce or something I didn't have in the pantry. Preparation was the key, as very little of my diet was available off the shelf. Two weeks in, and I already knew I was changing for the better. I was sleeping more soundly, my daily aches and pains were far less, and I had more energy. The bonus was I had yet to need my prescription medication for asthma. It was gone! No wheezing, no coughing, and no prescription drugs. With these successes, I did more digging. As the months rolled by, I finally stopped losing weight and settled approximately twenty pounds less. I had to buy clothes that actually fit me, and in fact had to replace most of my wardrobe.

After a lot more research, I settled on a grain-free, dairy-free and much-reduced-sugar diet using honey and pure maple syrup as sweeteners. I eventually got the hang of planning and preparation. I plan my meals and snacks a week in advance and always have something on hand to eat just in case.

Another few months went by and I still do not need asthma

medication. In addition, I used to have reflux occasionally, and this has not returned either. I recently went to a biometric screening for work insurance coverage. All the parameters they check were within normal limits, including lipids, blood pressure, and BMI. In other words, healthy.

At the end of the day, I would still rather change my diet than take toxic drugs, with their unknown and unpredictable-side effects, for the rest of my life. I still find it mind-boggling that some of my friends, acquaintances, and coworkers—and even my former gastrointestinal physician—would find it strange that I would not take prescription drugs for something that I believe can be controlled, or even cured, with diet modification. As stated previously, I have cured one chronic "disease" already and I am working on a few others. The future is uncertain. However, one thing I do know is that if I did not try, I would never know how much I can control versus relying on the "experts" to guide me.

Samantha's Story (Samantha's Words)

Patient: Samantha

Age: 27

Age when diagnosed with celiac disease: 16

Symptoms: Overweight, fatigued, lethargic, mood swings, depression, bed-wetting, underdeveloped bladder, anxiety, diarrhea, constipation, sharp stomach pains, gas, headaches, nausea, canker sores, delayed puberty, rashes, consistent tooth problems, heart arrhythmia, and frequent colds.

Family members diagnosed with celiac disease: Blood sister, half sister, half brother, cousins, great uncle and aunt, mom, grandfather, aunts and uncles.

The Diagnosis

I will never forget where I was when I realized my list of health concerns were anything but "normal." I was in a port-a-potty in the middle of Eastern Oregon, praying that I could actually go one day without having chronic diarrhea or constipation. I had taken a weeklong road trip with my friends, and although we were expecting to explore the beautiful sights of Oregon, we spent a majority of the time finding bathrooms and listening to my complaints about my horrible headaches and nasty stomach pains. After returning from the road, I made a trip into the doctor's office and essentially demanded an explanation. I wanted to know why I was sick, and what the doctors were going to do to make it better.

I was born a healthy baby with no apparent health issues. As an infant, I had very few health problems aside from a heart arrhythmia and an unexplained rash. The doctors informed my parents that the rash was no concern and I would grow out of the arrhythmia. Growing up, I was a fairly normal kid. I grew up on a farm south of Corvallis, and was raised by my dad. I spent most of my childhood playing in the fields with my sister and cousin.

However, my sister and I also spent a lot of time inside the house, sick with various flus and colds. I was sick throughout a large portion of elementary school. In the third grade, I missed a month of school because I was sick with a cold that just wouldn't go away. My weight was becoming a problem. I had previously been a fairly small child, but I started to gain weight that refused to come off. I also had horrible bladder problems and was a constant bed wetter. My doctor didn't think much of my weight or flu problems, and prescribed medication for my "underdeveloped" bladder. Another large portion of my childhood was spent in the dentist's office. Genetically, my whole family had bad teeth, so it was only standard that I would make monthly visits to the dentist.

I made it through my middle school years with very few problems, and it wasn't until high school that my health issues became more prevalent. I started to have problems at home. I had become extremely moody, depressed, and irritable. My dad and stepmom had a hard time dealing with me, but just assumed that I was a difficult teenager. At this point, I was obese and anxious, and had become extremely shy. I had also begun to realize how irregular my bowel movements were, and at the age of fourteen, I was still wetting the bed. Going to the doctor for my annual checkup, I expressed all my health concerns and poured my heart out about my depression and anxiety. My doctor decided it would be best to put me on an antidepressant and told me that otherwise he had no concerns.

As I began to move my way through high school, I put my issues aside and focused on doing well in school. I continued to have the same health concerns, and developed a few more. I started to have stomach pains, I was fatigued, I had constant headaches, I had a mysterious itchy rash on my knee, and I had not started my "cycle." My doctor decided that the majority of my problems were developing from being overweight, and that my headaches were due to my need to wear eyeglasses. He referred me to an optometrist and recommended I start watching my diet and working out. This would be the last time that I saw this doctor.

While I was having my own health concerns, my sister was having severe health problems of her own. My sister, Mary, had also suffered from health issues her entire life. Unfortunately, hers were much more severe and prevalent than mine. Mary was overweight, often had flu symptoms, and had chronic back pains, stomach pains, chronic diarrhea, and a long list of other problems. When our family practitioner dismissed her back and stomach pains, my parents decided to take Mary to the emergency room. Within hours of being in the ER, the cause of Mary's chronic pain had been discovered. She had a twenty-pound benign tumor in her abdomen that had wrapped itself around one of her ovaries and was continuing to grow. After removing the tumor, Mary made a slow recovery, but still continued to have persistent health problems. After seeing several different doctors and specialists, and developing several new health issues, Mary was finally diagnosed with celiac disease.

Knowing that our previous family doctor had severely misdiagnosed Mary, our whole family began to see a new doctor. After returning from my weeklong excursion with my friends, I marched into this doctor's office and demanded answers. To my surprise, he listened to me, took notes, asked questions, and looked for answers. Although he had not been the doctor to diagnose my sister, this doctor knew celiac disease was a genetic disorder and decided to do a blood test.

One week later, in September of 2004, I was diagnosed with celiac disease. In the following year, I began to turn my life around. However, attempting to become 100 percent gluten free was anything but easy. When I was first diagnosed, there were no gluten-free bakeries, there was little to no selection of gluten-free products in the store, and eating at restaurants was near impossible. I was overwhelmed with how to grocery shop, how to eat, and how to go on living a normal life. Unfortunately, my insurance would not cover a nutritionist or specialist, and my family could not afford to send me to one, so I started research on my own. I went to the library and searched for hours on the web and I started my journey to being gluten free.

Gluten Free... Right?

Within weeks of starting a gluten-free diet, I began to have normal bowel movements, my mood was improving, my headaches were disappearing, and I was finally beginning to lose weight. Well, as far as I was concerned, I was on a gluten-free diet—little did I know that every day I was continuing to harm my body. In January of 2005, I started my first job at a local pizza shop. I would continue to work at this pizza shop for the next six years of my life. My first year working was also my first year being gluten free. I remember feeling like I could do anything; most of my symptoms had gone away. I was finally healthy, I had friends, my energy was improving, and best of all, I had lost almost one hundred pounds.

It wasn't until 2007 that I realized my job could be causing health issues. I was feeling sick quite often, and I had horrible nausea, sharp pains in my chest, a rash on my hands, mood swings, canker sores, and continuing teeth complications. When I developed the rash on my hands, I decided to go to the doctor. I told him about my nausea and sharp pains, and I showed him the rash on my hands. He ordered a pregnancy test (for the nausea) and told me that the pizza shop could NOT be making me sick. He explained that gluten had to be ingested, and that while I was around gluten I wasn't ingesting it so it couldn't possibly be harming me. I was told that if I wanted proof, then I could have the endoscopy test done. I agreed and we went ahead with the test.

Five hundred dollars later, I still had no results. My doctor informed me that the camera revealed I was fine. He told me to write down everything I ate, and if I continued to feel sick, to come back and see him in six months. After talking to my family, I decided maybe I was being silly and perhaps this is how I was supposed to feel. This is when I realized that maybe I was never going to feel 100 percent, and I might spend the rest of my life feeling less than average.

Over the next three years, I continued to have persistent health problems. Although I knew my doctors and family thought I was a hypochondriac, I still continued to make various trips to the doctors for all different reasons. I was given all types of tests and blood work for all different diseases and ailments. I complained of constant nausea and sharp stomach pains. So I was given several different pregnancy tests, stool tests, and ultrasounds. Then when they couldn't find a problem I was prescribed medication to ease my pain. I felt fatigued and tired all the time, so they took my blood work for anemia and thyroid problems. When those came back negative, I was told to exercise more and stress less. I had severe mood swings and irritability, so I was told that I was on the wrong type of birth control and was put on several different types. I had severe sores on every part of my body, so I was tested for herpes… four times. When they finally ruled out herpes, I was given an ointment to put on the sores to ease the pain. I was also told that I had mono, heartburn, nerve damage, and stress headaches. It seemed that every doctor had a "treatment" for my problems. However, I didn't want a "treatment"—I wanted a solution. I was tired of wasting my time and money on doctors who weren't vested in truly making me feel better.

It was 2010 when I finally realized that my doctors were not going to be my advocate and I had to take my health into my own hands if I wanted to get better. I decided to forget everything my doctors had said, and I turned to forums and blogs on the Internet. This is where I discovered the overwhelming consensus that not only were my symptoms related to celiac disease, they were most likely a direct result of my daily exposure to gluten through work.

Of course, at this point, I was outraged. I knew what was making me sick, and I realized I had no idea how much damage had been done to my body over the past six years. I decided the best thing I could do was move forward, and I took every precaution I could. While I was at work, I wore masks and gloves, and I didn't touch any loose flour, but my symptoms were still present and only seeming to get worse. Unfortunately, finding a new job was not an easy task. I had worked at the same place for six years. My job had become a part of who I was. I developed a strong relationship with my boss, and she had invested a lot into developing me as her manager. However, I knew that my quality of life could be dramatically changed if I was able to find a new job. Shortly after I started my job search, I was lucky enough to find an opening to work at the Gluten Free RN office. Luckily, I was rescued from my gluten-filled job and started on my true gluten-free journey.

Fast-forward to today, I am a healthy twenty-seven-year-old and my entire house, including my husband, is gluten free. We have also been Paleo since the spring of 2011. Remaining on a diet of whole foods, limiting processed foods, and eliminating grains and dairy has truly made a remarkable difference in my health. I try to live by the "80/20" rule and eat mostly Paleo. As a result, I am the healthiest I have ever been. I rarely get sick, I no longer suffer from mysterious ailments, and I recently gave birth to a full-term, beautiful baby boy. Most of my family members have also realized that they have health issues that stem from gluten, and most of them have gone gluten free or Paleo as well. Going gluten free truly changed my life, and I feel extremely blessed that I have the opportunity to help others, including my children, understand that food truly is medicine.

Beth's Story (Beth's Words)

I was diagnosed with MS and Lyme ten years ago. I lost eyesight in one eye over eight times and had lesions on my eye nerves. A total of seventeen lesions in my brain and spine on last count. I lost all feeling in my legs and walked with a cane for a year. I rarely ever wanted to get out of bed and enjoy life. I had given up.

The doctor's best advice was to learn to live with it happily! Life is all about attitude, right? NO! I wanted to feel good too. I was not me anymore. I was a shell of a once-happy person. I had heard doctors say a healthy diet may help me feel better. It seemed silly to me—how could food do anything if their great drugs did nothing?

I loved my SAD (Standard American Diet). I dipped everything in ranch and washed it down with a Coke. I thought the joy my taste buds felt also made me feel good. Boy, was I wrong. That food had left me so inflamed.

I went and saw a very alternative practitioner who studies iridology. She looked in my eyes and said, "This will be easy. You just need good digestion and detox." She said, "You just need to feed your body the most nutritious food and your immune system will kick back on and you will be fine."

That was two years ago. By the way, I did not believe her at all!

I went vegetarian in the beginning. We did a big ten-day cleanse and I started to feel normal again. There was a glimmer of hope. But something was still missing. I randomly saw a video on Facebook about a doctor with MS. My mom's friend had been diagnosed recently so we hit play.

The first thing to pop on the screen: "Recorded on 11/11/11." Me and my bestie love 11/11 in all forms. It is our thing. I knew this video was going to be good. By the way, our other new thing is Lyme disease—we both test CDC positive. What is the likelihood of that? Especially in Oregon where they say we do not have Lyme disease. That is a whole other story.

Dr. Wahls has PPMS. That is the bad MS: primary progressive. I have RRMS, relapsing remitting, meaning it comes and goes, and you will have good months and bad months. Mine always seemed to be bad and worse months. But with PPMS, it is just downhill, no recovery. There is no treatment or cure for it.

In the video, she talks about taking all the best MS drugs and having the best doctors. Yet she was always getting sicker. She then decided to research the disease herself. She realized she needed to heal her mitochondria. She found the nutrients the mitochondria needed to heal. She supplemented with vitamins and it did not work. So she decided to find them in her food. This was how she developed the Wahls Paleo Diet.

She is now no longer in a wheelchair. She is biking 18 miles again and just started jogging again this year. She is my hero! Right now she has clinical trials treating MS with a Paleo diet. A clinical trial using REAL FOOD as medicine—that is unheard of. And guess what, first round was successful in treating fatigue, a major problem for people with MS. She is going to change the world, and I am going to help!

Shopping a couple weeks later, I saw a Paleo bar in the store, made by a local Oregon company, Paleo Eats. It was so good, that I said, "I can do this! I am going Paleo!" I asked the owner, Debbie, on Facebook what book I should buy, and she suggested Practical Paleo by Diane Sanfilippo, BS, NC. I ordered it on

Amazon. The book came as we were walking out the door to visit the in-laws in Texas. I threw it in my carry-on and boarded the plane.

The first words in the book: *"Let food be thy medicine, and medicine be thy food." —Hippocrates.*

Diane writes, "Know this: We are not smarter than nature. We cannot make better food than nature. We need to eat real, whole food—period."

I was in love. Diane's book spoke to me as she broke down what the grains and the dairy were doing to my body. Something clicked for me, and I jumped right in. I instantly gave up all grains/dairy/legumes/soy/corn that day and added back in organic pastured animal products. It was very easy to find great grass-fed beef in Texas!

It just so happens by following this diet and only buying organic and mostly local ingredients we cut out all GMOs from our diet. We do not even eat meat that eats GMO feed. We take this seriously. It is not a diet; it is a lifestyle I love and embrace!

That was August 10, 2013. Result: I have been in remission from my MS and Lyme disease since December 2013. It took less than four months of getting the GMOs out of my diet for my autoimmune disease to shut off. And I lost eighty pounds! Just a huge bonus!

I am walking up hills again! Volunteering in our local food movement because I have the energy. I am a new, happy, healthier version of me. I love me again! You really learn to appreciate life when it is so close to gone.

Tiffanee's Story (Tiffanee's Words)

My name is Tiffanee Crowson, I am going to share my story. I am 38 I was raised in small town Monroe between Eugene & Corvallis a non-church home so I didn't attend church on a regular basis. I was 14 when I was a freshman in high school. Made it through my 4 treacherous years of high school where I got teased. Laughed @ made fun of when I tried out for sports, became the manager I Didn't have many friends through my 4 years of high school. Hung out by myself a lot when I was a junior/senior in high school I wanted to commit suicide when I was in love with this guy a year ahead of me didn't pay attention to me. My parents split up my senior year. I lived at different friends house form time to time after my high school graduation. I attended this class on the campus with developmentally challenged young adults. I was the top person in the class. I have lived on my own since I was about 17 years old in Corvallis where I attended class every day to learn how to wash my clothes, cook for myself, plan meals for myself. I did that until I was twenty one. Graduated and have lived independently since. I started attending NW Hills some time ago, my friend Sheryl told me of a group called Young Singles Group. I was egotistic @first i thought ok I will show up here is my chance I will meet a guy for sure, I thought it was a dating service so I showed up the first day I apparently missed it so I showed up the next day and I walk in and they are reading the bible and talking to one another I was like okay so this isn't a dating young singles group oh well I will stay and bear it that is where I met Jenny B. She introduced me to some people like Melanie, Eric, Chris and Amy they helped me along the way after I realized it wasn't a dating service I really enjoyed it going every Tuesday night I went for a few months/years then it ended in between that I worked @ Albertsons 4 1/2 years I learned a lot their I should have been let go many of times but through the good, bad & ugly I fought tooth and nail to go back I always ended up going back with a fake smile but I became a better person for it taught me a lot to grow up & be a better person. In 2009/2010 I met this wonderful role model idol influence mentor her name is Kim. She happened to be in the store on this particular day where I was having problems with my stomach. That day she had mentioned to me I should come down to her office & see the Gluten Free RN. I kept putting it off until this time I saw Kim again @ the store she asked me again if I was coming she said jokingly if you don't comedown I will tie you with a rope and drag you myself. WE both laughed. She gave me her phone number. I called her and went down and saw my other wonderful role model idol mentor influence Nadine Grzeskowiak. I found out about celiac disease, went on a gluten free diet, still have a few problems but for the most part better. These are two of the biggest influences in my life ever. They saw me for who I really am. The what ifs come in to play a big part in that. I was still employed @ Albertson's after a few months of that Albertsons went out of business so I was out of a job until I got the luck of the draw I got a job @ OSU which I thought was a dream job but it didn't turn out to what I thought. Then again my great friend, Kim typed out my resume turned it in to the office, which I thought was going to be working for the OSU Football team ended up not working out. I was a ticket taker for the games that ended soon. Then I had nowhere to turn I was out of a job, had nothing going on for me but my 2 biggest influences were still there for me, Nadine Grzeskowiak and Kim Heede just when I would lose Hope Nadine would send me a text to tell me there is something better, just be patient& wait. Then in April/March, Kim mentioned to me this place called G3 Sports & Fitness. I had mentioned this to my job coach who works with people with developmental disabilities. I said my good friend mentioned this place called G3. He kind of laughed it off then one day he was like okay we will go check it out. They loved me! I kept checking back in periodically without telling my job coach, Kirk. I would drive by and just look at it then drive away then almost towards the end of 2013 I went back again and I got offered a job. I started my first day out there was May 27th. I sanitize the weight room equipment, clean the bathrooms, vacuum, work out a little bit of everything I can. I can honestly say, without my two biggest influences who will remain in my life forever. I don't know where I would be without them. I am as happy as a lark still employed at G3, love every minute of it. I think where god intervened in my life is on the ninth of July I was leaving work @ 10:00 @ nite. I was on hwy 99 coming back from G3 sports. A bug had flown in my car, which I thought was a bug, it ended up being a bee and I am allergic to them so I got stung as I was on hwy 99 no where to pull over. I made it to Safeway where I went inside and fell over got some help & sat there for a while then left between leaving G3 & going to Safeway I don't remember how I made it to there really all I want in life is just a chance with some Gr8 guy that is into sports& can drive & melt my butter. I have been let down so many times I just want to find the right dude that is tough enuff 2 climb all the way to the top of a tree for an apple aka as falling & getting hurt cause once U have me I will never let you down I am A Gr* person friend GF jock shorts fit sun of a Aviator glasses my hair persice puka shell Blonde highlights dress 2 be comfortable aka hanes shirt with shorts & tan legs cute face or Vneck white shirt converse check girly girl!!!!!!:} just ask NADINE GRZESKOWIAK!!!!!!!! In the midst of all my celiac disease I had stage 4 liver failure & I remarkably got better with going GLUTEN FREE NADINE GRZESKOWIAK

IS MY ROCK. HERO. IDOL. I LOVE HER TOO PIECES WITH EVERY BONE IN MY BODY I WOULD GO TO HELL & BACK 4 HER!!!!!!!! LOVE U ROCK***

Tiffanee's Story (Nadine's Words)

Back in August of 2011, Kim mentioned that there would be this woman that would be coming to the office, and would I mind seeing if I could help her? Her concern was genuine and valid. When Tiffanee first came into the Gluten Free RN office, I introduced myself and sat down to hear a bit of Tiffanee's story as told by Tiffanee.

Tiffanee has Williams Syndrome, which is a genetic condition. In Dr. Oliver Sacks' book *Musicophilia,* he notes that people with Williams syndrome seem to be very musically inclined. I excitedly asked Tiffanee if she played instruments or had an incredible singing voice.

She responded, "Hell no. I like sports: football, baseball, basketball."

I am still not convinced Tiffanee is not some undiscovered musical prodigy, so I keep bugging her to pick up instruments or sing along with the radio. I drive her crazy, but I am undeterred. Tiffanee is adamant that she only likes sports, and she lives and dies for every one of the Oregon State University sports teams.

I had recently given a class on the increased rate of celiac disease in people with Down, Turner and Williams syndromes; by some reports, as much as 50 percent of the people in these populations test positive for the anti-gliadin antibodies (AGA). All of the studies I referenced for my talk strongly recommended these people get tested every year for celiac disease.

Tiffanee, though, had never been tested. She told me that some of the men she worked with at the grocery store were asking her when her baby was due. One of them actually asked her if she was having twins. I asked if she was pregnant and she gave me one of those "No way in hell" looks, which, of course, I had seen before and not necessarily believed. Tiffanee related her health issues, which included stage four liver failure, which led to the fluid retention or ascites that made her look as if she might be pregnant, which she wasn't. She stated she had Budd-Chiari Syndrome, which causes blood clots that can block the hepatic veins, the blood vessels that take blood from the liver. Tiffanee had also endured a traumatic abdominal injury while playing basketball in a tournament. Her doctors were waiting for the occlusion of her hepatic vessels to get bad enough, and the plan was for surgery. Tiffanee also had splenomegaly, she was severely anemic, she was a diabetic with a reported HbA1C of 11.2, her hands were cracked and bleeding, and she had a host of other significant medical issues.

After requesting that Tiffanee's primary care providers test her for celiac disease and gluten intolerance, she came to my "Intro to Gluten Intolerance and Celiac Disease" class. Then she and I went shopping for gluten-free foods that would be easy for her to prepare but still nutrient dense. Tiffanee learned the basics of a gluten-free diet very quickly. If someone tells me that shopping for gluten-free food and going gluten free is too hard, I always recommend Tiffanee as a great teacher.

Within a very short period of time on a gluten-free diet, her medical reports were coming back as "significantly improved," "may not need this medication anymore," and "no longer has liver failure," and her HbA1C has consistently been between 5.4 and 5.9 (with the normal range between 4.0 and 6.0).

Tiffanee's health has improved in remarkable and indisputable ways. Tiffanee is one of my heroes and truly pays attention to every word I say. I have to be careful sometimes. I am very proud of Tiffanee and her stalwart resolve to live gluten free for her continued health. Not only is the ascites significantly improved now that she no longer suffers from stage four liver failure, her anemia is resolving, and she no longer is facing a life-threatening surgery in a compromised state.

Tiffanee is now working on her "six-pack"! She wants washboard abs like our friend, Cain Credicott, whom she lovingly refers to as "Ab Man." Nothing would make Tiffanee happier than a photo of

Cain and his abs. (Hint hint, Cain!)

My job as a nurse is to recognize a sick person and act appropriately. As a registered nurse, I take my duty as a patient advocate very seriously, especially when working with anyone within a vulnerable population. Some days, I think that is all of us.

Conclusion

Several years ago, when I was beginning to educate myself, I asked if I could pick the brain of a wheat scientist I had met at a party. This person—let's call him or her Wheaty—said he/she would meet with me, but it had to be off campus, in the back of a coffee shop, and off the record. After Wheaty had retired, he/she would speak to me on the record. What?!? Wheaty told me that if he/she were to be seen speaking with me, he/she would be fired. Seriously? Wow.

We did have a couple of meetings in the backs of coffee shops off campus, and I learned quite a bit about the science of wheat, though not enough to be a wheat expert by any stretch of the imagination. When I told Wheaty that the University of Washington had received a grant to develop a "gluten-free wheat," he/she laughed and said that would never happen.

I pulled out the article in the paper that stated as much, and Wheaty's response was, "I am sure they were happy to get that money, but they know it will never happen. You can't take the gluten out of wheat; it's not possible." From the mouth of a wheat scientist.

Celiac disease is not just about health. It is a social, political, and economic issue of great importance, on an individual, family, city, state, national, and international level. When I would send letters to former Governor Kitzhaber about front-page articles in the Oregonian related to state spending for health care for the 20 percent of Oregon's population that uses 80 percent of our health-care dollars, I usually made bold requests suggesting he should give those patients to me. I would love to have them tested for celiac disease and gluten intolerance, change their diet, and see the difference it will make for them as individuals and in our state's health-care spending. It sounds so easy, says I, the nurse.

But the reality is that Oregon grows lots and lots of wheat. Much of our state economy is based on the commodity of wheat on the national and world market. Oregon State University, located where

I live in Corvallis, was even credited with hybridizing wheat so it is shorter, disease resistant, and grows really well in Oregon. After contacting several of my elected officials directly through letters and phone calls, as well as attempting to get grants and state government contracts as a woman running a small business, I realized that they always had someone to punt me to, but nothing fruitful ever came out of these contacts. Dead ends. It is conceivable that given the political and economic aspects of living in a state that grows megatons of wheat, continuing to bury the facts surrounding celiac disease might sound like a good idea.[2]

My stance always comes back to the fact that we will fail in our efforts to save health-care dollars until we recognize gluten intolerance and celiac disease as significant issues that have been ignored for over seventy years in the United States. Can you imagine where our health-care system would be if we had failed to recognize type 1 or insulin-dependent diabetes mellitus (IDDM) as a health issue, and only treated the symptoms? There is significant genetic overlap between IDDM and celiac disease. All of the pediatric endocrinology centers across the United States test every child with IDDM for celiac disease every year, because these kids are at increased risk for celiac disease, and because they may seroconvert at any time. But we as a nation do not routinely test every IDDM adult, typically even once, let alone every year.

Meanwhile, type 2 or non-insulin-dependent diabetes is not considered to be autoimmune, but it *is* related to being overweight—it's a diet-related health problem, as is gluten intolerance. But while we recognize type 2 diabetes as an enormous public health issue, we as a nation are just now beginning to recognize gluten intolerance and celiac disease as "real" medical problems.

Interestingly, because there is a recognized genetic overlap between IDDM and celiac disease, if we are collectively failing to recognize celiac disease, then it will be even more difficult to manage all of the diabetic patients rapidly coming down the pike. Can you begin to see why this is such an enormous public health crisis? It is currently estimated that 50 percent of the United States

2. That said, (now former) Governor Kitzhaber, who is a physician himself, has been very progressive in forming the Archimedes Movement toward a single payer system that follows a coordinated care organization or CCO method of health-care delivery.

population will have some form of diabetes by 2050. Do you know who is excited about that figure? The pharmaceutical companies and the corporations that sell all of those diabetic supplies. What a market. What a scam. It is also estimated that this generation of children will not live past the age of us, their parents. They will die at a younger age. We as a country are sliding backwards on the scales of health and longevity.

Of course, there is also the concept that once you have one autoimmune disease, the chance of developing another one is 30 to 50 percent greater than for someone in the "normal" population. Now, I have been on the lookout for the "normal" population, and I just haven't gotten a good grasp on whom that might be.

I also call into serious question the idea that celiac disease should even be considered an "autoimmune" disease. There is no other autoimmune disease—or disease, period—that potentially presents with 300-plus signs and symptoms. The theory I am working on that suggests the damage caused by gluten grains is a poisoning and not an autoimmune reaction. What if all of these people with multiple sclerosis, amyloidosis, lupus, Sjögren's, insulin-dependent diabetes, vitiligo, Raynaud's, and the list goes on, started out with celiac disease or by being gradually poisoned by gluten-containing grains? Because we are not testing most Americans for celiac disease first, doesn't it make sense that there is a distinct possibility that most of those autoimmune diseases could be at least in part triggered by the continued consumption of wheat, barley, rye, and oats? It is ludicrous to suggest that failing to recognize gluten intolerance and celiac disease for at least over sixty years is not at least partly to blame for the current epidemic of autoimmune diseases.

None of this is about selling you anything. The information is all here and there. If you are inclined to look up the myriad of research articles from around the world, please use both the c-e-l-i-a-c spelling and the c-o-e-l-i-a-c spelling; you will get more diverse research articles from around the world. When I am in the process of vetting a research article, I want to know who paid for the research. Is the research related to a pharmaceutical company? Are the researchers being paid by a pharmaceutical company?

Who stands to benefit financially from the research results as they are presented? Do I trust the doctors and researchers that are named as the research team based on hearing them present at celiac conferences, or is the material they typically present biased because they are taking money and/or perks from pharmaceutical corporations?

What I find most interesting is that instead of flooding the media with EVERYONE MUST GET TESTED FOR CELIAC DISEASE BECAUSE THE UNITED STATES FORGOT TO TEST PEOPLE FOR OVER SEVENTY YEARS, the celiac experts have been busy developing a non-dietary treatment plan, a pill that will never work as well as a gluten-free diet does, so that there is something for people to buy. There is an enormous amount of international pressure to come up with a pill, vaccine, or something to SELL. Otherwise, it is just a diet change and people get better. Make no mistake: this is the largest untapped market in the world.

Shortly after officially starting the Gluten Free RN in 2007, I started blogging about our experiences. One of my first blog posts was entitled "Questions That Need Answers Regarding Celiac Disease," and it detailed the burning questions on my mind after my initial research into celiac disease.

1. Why isn't there one study in the whole country on the incidence of celiac disease in the Native American population? A PubMed search of this question came back with no published research data and no current studies in progress. How can this be?

2. I have offered to give presentations or in-services (classes) to every physician group I know. Not one physician group has taken me up on that offer? Why not?

3. How come in 2004 the National Institutes of Health (NIH) launched a celiac disease awareness campaign and no one heard about it? Not one health-care professional I have spoken to knows about this campaign. This is still a conundrum to me.

4. Why are physicians so sure that even if they *did* diagnose celiac disease, the diet is *so* hard, no one would follow it? I have had this conversation many times, with many doctors. One even professed to have tried the diet and failed.

5. Are Asian people at lower risk for celiac disease—or not? It used to be assumed that Asian people had a lower risk for celiac disease because they tend to be DQ4 gene carriers. But it has been determined that celiac disease may occur in the Asian population at the same rate as the rest of the world, especially now that Asia has adopted the standard American diet or SAD.

6. If the rate of celiac disease in Sub-Saharan Africa is 1 in 65, why are we feeding the starving children wheat?

7. Is anyone going to start telling African-Americans they may be at greater risk for celiac disease?

8. Why are the pharmaceutical companies spending millions of dollars to develop a pill for celiac disease? The treatment is a diet change.

9. How did an entire disease process known to the rest of the world get hidden by the United States for over 120 years?

10. Why is the media *so* slow to pick up this humiliating story and give it the coverage it deserves?

11. To the doctors: How many patients in your practice have you diagnosed with celiac disease?

12. To the nurses: I challenge you to be patient advocates and learn the symptoms of celiac disease.

Now, several years later, some of these questions now have at least partial answers, and I might rephrase a few of them—but for the most part they are unanswered, and the list has only gotten longer.

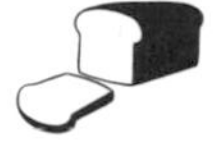

My immersion into the world of gluten intolerance and celiac disease began the minute I heard those two previously unknown phrases and has continued non-stop for the past eight years. My eyes and ears are always on laser alert for anything related to these topics. My office is located next to the Book Bin in Corvallis, and their friendly, quirky staff will often helpfully bring to my attention old and new books related to my specialty. One day several years ago, while cruising the aisles of the Book Bin, I saw a green book entitled *Good Food, Gluten Free: For those for whom "the staff of life" is slow poison—a world of safe nutrition,* written by a woman named Hilda Cherry Hills, a nutritionist. Two of the main reasons it caught my eye were 1) it was an older book, upon inspection written in 1976, and 2) on the back cover it read "My Daily/Deadly Bread," which appealed to my ex-Catholic heathen self. Hilda Cherry Hills wrote the first Paleo book in 1976. If there is one before then, I haven't found it yet.

I tried to do research on Hilda but came up with very little on the Internet. There is significantly more on her famous husband, Lawrence D. Hills, a well-regarded and accomplished English organic horticulturist who was a sickly child, was in a wheelchair for most of his adult life, and was restored to health and rescued from his wheelchair simply by changing his diet, thanks to—you guessed it—his wife, Hilda Cherry Hills. Her basic premise in *Good Food, Gluten Free* was, *Why would I feed my celiac husband crappy, nutrient-deficient grains and flours—or even more ghastly, wheat starch!—when I could feed him meats, veggies, fruits, nuts, and seeds, i.e. healthy foods?* Sounds Paleo to me! One of her other books is entitled *Good Food, Milk Free, Grain Free.* My hero.

I searched high and low to find out if she was still alive and living in England or somewhere else, but to no avail. It wasn't long after I had discovered Hilda's books and displayed them in my street-level office window, that one night after locking up and walking through the dark parking lot to my car, a man approached me, quite out of the shadows, and said, "Excuse me, do you know of Cherry? Cherry Hills?"

"No, I don't know that person," I responded, caught off guard and not sure who this man was.

"Are you sure?" he said, "Hilda Cherry Hills. The woman who wrote those books in the window of your office. I lived with her and her husband, Lawrence, in England."

I was stunned and elated that someone who knew the object of my fascination and research was approaching me and offering up firsthand knowledge on one of my idols! Jeremy had lived with and worked with Lawrence and Cherry Hills in England, and now he was living in Corvallis, Oregon. How does this happen?! Amazing. Jeremy is a brilliant mathematician and genius artist, and he and I have had several meetings about Cherry. Jeremy has shared photos, news articles, and stories of his personal interactions with the now-deceased Hilda Cherry Hills.

One of the members of our support group came into my office one day, somewhat distraught, and asked me, "Do I have to kill myself? Because if I have to go live in one of those assisted living facilities, they will kill me anyway. There is no way they can feed me gluten free! They all say they can't offer or guarantee that anything is gluten free. That's not living. I would rather be dead than have to be paranoid about every meal I was eating in one of those places."

That particular conversation led to some brainstorming sessions about what WE would need and want in such a facility. We talked about the idea of a place that is totally gluten free, with a strong emphasis on the Paleo lifestyle. A place where newly diagnosed celiac patients can come with their families, live for six to eight weeks in a gluten-free bubble, get detoxed, learn how to make food choices and why, and begin the healing process. The other component of the facility is a gluten-free long-term care side where celiac people can come to live as they age.

Handily, I had already been planning for years something along the same lines for retired nurses. In an effort to honor Hilda Cherry Hills, whom I am certain I would have absolutely adored had we met, I have intentions of naming the facility I have patented after her. *H. Cherry Hills Rehab and Long Term Care, where food is incredibly tasty and healthy and life is very good.*

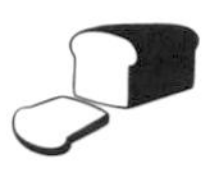

I wish someone had told me when I was first diagnosed what I have now told you. I am a cut-to-the-chase kind of person. I don't like to waste time, energy, or money. Well, money I will "waste" if it's on something fun, like food, travel, yarn, more food, books, and more travel. But doctors, prescription medications, and time wasted chasing phantom diagnoses—not so much. It has certainly been a journey that has challenged me to the core of who I am as a person, as a mother, as a nurse, and as a patient advocate. I've had to redefine myself in each of those roles.

In a nutshell, I do this work and I write this book, because there was no one like me who I could have gone to for help when I needed it most. After I was diagnosed (and then not diagnosed), I saw a montage of random practitioners who could and did help me up to a certain point—and then I had to keep searching and learning, and eventually had to relearn everything I had been taught. Everything I had been taught about medicine, nursing, food, being a mother, health, and healing was wrong. Not just for me, but for my family, my friends, my friends' families, and my patients. I carried guilt (raised Catholic, go figure) for a long time because it was my job to know, and I didn't know. A friend asked me why I gave up my career as an agency nurse specializing in emergency nursing that paid at least $75 an hour. He told me most people thought I was completely crazy. Whacked. I had lost my mind, they said.

The fact is I almost did lose my mind and my body, along with my soul. Death nearly got a hold of me. By all rights, I should be dead.

But I am not dead. I lived. I am still recovering, and my body is damaged, no doubt about it. It was horrible to stand in the shower with my failing body, day after torturous day, and as a nurse, not be able to self-diagnose. Maddening, actually, enough to make me lose my mind. But I didn't lose my mind. I got it back, along with my body, my health, and my strength.

I honestly have no choice but to do this work. This work needs to be done so that others don't have to suffer and die needlessly. My whole life has prepared me for this job. Once you know something is true and you experience a true paradigm shift, you can't go back and pretend you don't know anymore. At least I can't pretend I don't know. The deniers will always be present and accounted for, which is great. What I see in public and professionally leads me to believe the people that are the biggest defenders of grains are the most addicted and the most ill-affected. I hope for their sake and their families' sake, despite their rabid defense of wheat, barley, rye, oats and all other grains, that they remain healthy and happy.

I often ask myself, how many lives do I have to touch, influence or attempt to change before my "work" is done? Will my work ever be done? What am I fighting? What am I fighting *for*? Why do I even give a shit? Overwhelmingly, I fight for my young self and all of those other children who struggle to survive in chaos and dysfunction, and sometimes, hell. I can most assuredly manage chaos, and I manage it well. Chaos is my life. Chaos ruled my childhood, it ruled the emergency departments, and it still rules generally throughout my life. In my struggle for peace and quiet, I have embraced the challenges and struggles, and have even been drawn to the chaos. What has always kept me going was the illusion that there was peace and quiet and calm just around the bend, if only I worked hard enough. If only I sacrificed enough. If only I WAS enough. That peace has eluded me and continues to elude me to this day.

One last question I would like you to ponder: Why do we run from the truth? Are we incapable of incorporating the truth until we ourselves experience a catastrophic event? I would have been so grateful if someone, anyone had pulled me aside and said, *I see that you are suffering with [whatever symptom I was demonstrating that day]. You might have an issue with wheat or gluten. Even if you get tested and the test is negative, go gluten free and see if you feel better. You have nothing to lose, except those symptoms, that weight, and that skin rash.*

It is always easier to maintain good health than it is to regain it. Our bodies are remarkable in their ability to compensate and keep all their systems working despite being stressed, malnourished, and poisoned. But at some point, we may all hit that tipping point into the abyss of illness or death. I hope you will be inspired to investigate, research, and find the path that makes you feel amazing and provides you with a long and happy life devoid of disease. Everything you are exposed to has the ability to turn on or turn off genes. It's called epigenetics. We should not assume our bodies are supposed to fall apart, that our brains have to shrink as we age, that our bones must become fragile, or that we're bound to develop any of those "familial" diseases. *Aging* is normal. Dying of preventable diseases is not.

References

1. Catassi, Carlo, Ilse-Maria Ràtsch, Lenora Gandolfi, Riccardo Pratesi, Elisabetta Fabiani, Ramzi El Asmar, Maria Frijia, Italo Bearzi, and Luciano Vizzoni. "Why is coeliac disease endemic in the people of the Sahara?" *The Lancet* 354, no. 9179 (1999): 647–648.
2. Fasano, Alessio. "Where Have All the American Celiacs Gone?" *Acta Paediatrica* 412 (1996): 20–24.
3. Fry, Lionel, MD. "What Is DH?" *Crossed Grain*, Summer 2001, reprinted with permission on the Dermatitis Herpetiformis Online Community, http://www.dermatitisherpetiformis.org.uk/index.html (accessed May 22, 2015)
4. Gee, Samuel. "On the Cœliac Affection," *St Bart's Hosp Rep*. 1888;24:17–20.
5. Green, Peter H. R., and Rory Jones. *Celiac Disease: A Hidden Epidemic*. New York: Collins, 2006.
6. Green, Peter H. R., Alfred I. Neugut Afzal J. Naiyer, Z. Collette Edwards, Susan Gabinelle, and Vijit Chinburapa. "Economic Benefits of Increased Diagnosis of Celiac Disease in a National Managed Care Population in the United States." *J Insur Med* 40, no. 3 4 (2008): 218–228.
7. Greszkowiak, Nadine. "Questions That Need Answers Regarding Celiac Disease," *Gluten Free RN*, April 19, 2008, http://glutenfreern.com/questions-that-need-answers-regarding-celiac-disease/.
8. Groopman, Jerome E. *How Doctors Think*. Boston: Houghton Mifflin, 2007.
9. Haas, Sidney V., and Merrill Patterson Haas. *Management of Celiac Disease*. Philadelphia: Lippincott, 1951.
10. Hills, Hilda Cherry. *Good Food, Gluten Free*. New Canaan, Conn.: Keats Pub., 1976.
11. Hills, Hilda Cherry. *Good Food, Milk Free, Grain Free*. Health Science ed. New Canaan, Conn.: Keats Pub., 1980.

12. Libonati, Cleo J. *Recognizing Celiac Disease: Signs, Symptoms, Associated Disorders & Complications*. Fort Washington, Pa.: Gluten Free Works Pub., 2007.
13. "Celiac Disease Is Treated Without the Banana Diet." *The New York Times*, October 4, 1942.
14. "'Celiac Disease': Most Children Are Now Cured But Cause Is Still Unknown." *The New York Times*, May 21, 1950.
15. Stenberg, Reidun, Marios Hadjivassiliou, Pascale Aeschlimann, Nigel Hoggard, and Daniel Aeschlimann. "Anti-Transglutaminase 6 Antibodies in Children and Young Adults with Cerebral Palsy." *Autoimmune Diseases* 2014 (2014): 1–8. doi:10.1155/2014/237107.

C-reactive protein <30
1.8
Creatine Kinase
46 (28 181)